Linda,

Hope you enjoy the reading.

All my best,
Erica

Handbook of Leads for
Pacing, Defibrillation
& Cardiac Resynchronization

Acknowledgements

I would like to thank my family, friends and colleagues around the world for their continuous affection, support and encouragement. My sincere gratitude to all of you.

I also would like to convey my appreciation to Medtronic, Inc. for their continued support over the years.

Handbook of Leads for Pacing, Defibrillation & Cardiac Resynchronization

Erick Cuvillier, MSc

© 2009 E. Cuvillier

All rights reserved. No part of this publication may be reproduced in any form or by any electronic or mechanical means, including information storage and retrieval systems, without permission in writing from the author, except by a reviewer who may quote brief passages in a review.

Unless otherwise indicated, all intellectual property rights in the photographs and drawings used herein are owned by Medtronic, Inc. and are used by the author with the express permission of Medtronic, Inc.

First published 2009
ISBN 978-1-59608-585-5

Printed in:
Imprenta Llorens, Inc.
Road 14 Km. 11.2, Juana Díaz, PR 00795
Tels. 787-837-4055 • 787-260-0407 • 787-837-0653

Contents

Foreword, vii

Introduction, ix

1 Historical Milestones, 1
Cardiac pacing, 1
Cardiac defibrillation, 8

2 Cardiovascular System, Cardiac Rhythm and Disorders, 13
Heart, 13
Electrical conduction system, 14
Heart beat anatomy, 15
Heart rhythm disorders, 16
Heart failure, 18

3 Pacing Lead Terminology and Technology, 23
Description of an implantable pacing system, 23
Construction and components, 24
Polarity, 26
Length and diameter, 29

4 Tachy Lead Terminology and Technology, 31
Description and implantable cardioverter defibrillator system, 31
Evolution of technology, 33
Construction and components, 36
Polarity, 41
Shocking circuits, 42
Coil electrode, 44

5 CRT Lead and Delivery System Terminology and Technology, 47
Description of an implantable biventricular pacing system, 47
Construction and components, 48
Delivery systems and fixation mechanisms, 49

6 Epimyocardial Lead Terminology and Technology, 57
Construction and components, 57
Applications, 59
Special tools required for implants, 59

7 Temporary Pacing Lead, 61
Construction and components, 61
Applications, 63

8 Electrode, 65
Fixation mechanisms, 65
Materials and designs, 68
Steroid, 72

9 Conductor, 75
Materials, 75
Designs and definitions, 77

10 Insulation, 81
Insulation materials, 81
Silicone, 81
Polyurethane, 82
Fluoropolymers, 84
Copolymers, 84
Properties of insulation materials, 86

11 Connector, 89
Designs and definitions, 89
Adaptors, 91

12 Stylet and Guide Wire, 93
Stylet, 93
Stylet guide, 95
Locking stylet, 95
Guide wire, 96

13 Suture Sleeve, 99

14 Fluorovisibility, 101
Equipment, 101
Views and interpretations, 101

15 Glossary, 105

16 Suggested Readings, 117

Foreword

"The past is a foreign country: they do things differently there."
L. P. Hartley (1895 – 1972) *The Go-Between.*

Travel is said to broaden the mind, but much of what has happened over the past 50 years of cardiac pacing would suggest the foreign country that is the past had become a single, sedentary global nation with regard to the pacing lead.

Until fairly recently, very few had questioned the traditions of lead design, construction and implant techniques despite a wealth of information being available from past experience. The result was that the pacing lead had become devalued while representing the weakest link in the pacing chain and being the part that gave the most problems for patient and health-care professional alike. The main concern was for the design of a thin lead that could be placed as quickly as possible, forgetting that the lead may have to function in a very hostile environment for the next 20 years or more.

In this book, the history of the pacing lead is analyzed in breadth and depth, and the lessons of history are re-examined to direct us towards the needs of delivering pacing therapy for the 21st century. Many will be surprised at how much effort has gone into trying to make this "simple wire" resistant to the attacks of time, the human body and the implanting clinician.

Enjoy the journey and discover how the past 50 years can inform the future – in the next half-century the conduit for delivering pacing therapy will undoubtedly undergo radical changes that will influence our practice of cardiac pacing and enable us to provide novel and more effective cardiac electrical therapy.

Michael Gammage, MD
University of Birmingham, United Kingdom

Introduction

"Ignorance is the night of the mind,
but a night without moon and star."
Confucius *Chinese philosopher & reformer* (551 BC - 479 BC)

Current implantable pacemakers owe their existence to the invention of external pacing devices. Their refinement is linked to several coincidental developments in such diverse fields as cardiovascular surgery, electrical engineering and polymer chemistry. Similarly, pacing leads have benefited from remarkable technological advances. Passive and active fixation mechanisms have become popular for use in the atrium and the ventricle. Hybrid insulation and new conductor materials have made leads thinner and more reliable. Electrodes are small, porous and steroid-eluting to optimize stimulation thresholds. Today's implanting physicians can also position the leads in nontraditional pacing sites using sophisticated delivery systems.

Leads are the electrical conduit between an implantable device and the heart. They transmit therapeutic energies to the cardiac tissue and return sensed information back to the electronic device for diagnostic and monitoring purposes. Leads must withstand an extremely harsh environment, permanently span multiple anatomical and physiological environments (Figure 1) and undergo approximately 400 million heartbeat-induced deformations over a 10-year period within the heart.

Figure 1. Anatomical regions commonly spanned by transvenous endocardial pacing leads.

A: Pocket
B: Clavicle / first rib
C: Venous
D: Intracardiac
E: Tissue interface

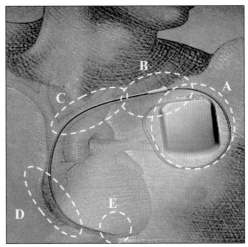

This textbook addresses the ongoing engineering challenges and critical design factors that allow leads to operate safely in the human heart. The readers will come across straightforward and self-explanatory illustrations for an easy to read and comprehensive overview of the subject.

As a final point, I welcome your comments on this first initiative and your suggestions for the future editions that will address ongoing technological developments and research findings.

Erick Cuvillier
erick.cuvillier@gmail.com

CHAPTER 1

Historical Milestones

Cardiac pacing

In the 1920s and 1930s, the pacing theory was for the first time translated into effective, yet limited, therapy. Working independently of one another, Dr. Mark Lidwell of Australia and Dr. Albert Hyman (Figure 1) of the United States developed external cardiac pacemakers for clinical application.

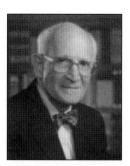

Figure 1. Dr. Albert Hyman

Lidwell described his portable device at a medical conference in Sydney in 1929; he reported that he had revived one infant after he applied an "electrically powered invention to the child's heart". Hyman, in New York City, NY, reported on his own pacing device in 1932. Unlike Lidwell's machine, which plugged into a wall socket and required "plunging" a needle into the patient's ventricle, Hyman's device was driven by a hand-cranked spring-wound motor (Figure 2) and provided electrical pulses to the right atrium via a needle electrode (Figure 3). Dr. Hyman faced considerable opposition from the medical and social community and never found a manufacturer for the device.

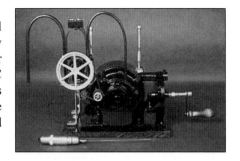

Figure 2. Hyman's "artificial cardiac pacemaker" operated by a hand crank and spring motor which turned a magnet (DC current generator). Electricity was introduced into the heart by a needle plunged through the chest wall and would cause the heart to beat.

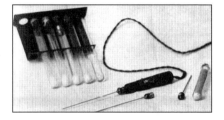

Figure 3. Electrical impulses were directed into the patient's right atrium through a bipolar needle electrode introduced via an intercostal space.

An external pacemaker developed in the early 1950s by Dr. Paul Zoll (Figure 4) brought happier results.

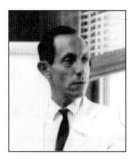

Figure 4. Dr. Paul Zoll

In November 1952, Zoll, an experienced cardiologist and researcher working at Beth Israel Hospital in Boston, MA, announced the resuscitation of a 65-year-old cardiac patient. Zoll's external pacemaker maintained the patient's heartbeat for more than 50 hours at a time, and the man recovered sufficiently to eventually go home.

The external pacemakers of the 1950s had several serious drawbacks. They were large and AC-powered devices that plugged into the wall and therefore necessitated extension cords. The AC requirement severely limited the patient's mobility and, more significantly, made the occasional power outage a potentially life-threatening event. They were also uncomfortable and traumatic for the patient, often burning the skin where the electrodes were attached to the chest (Figure 5).

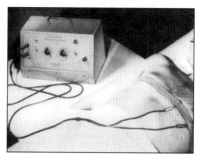

Figure 5. Dr. Zoll's external tabletop pacemaker. It delivered periodic electric impulses through a pair of metal electrodes strapped to the patient's chest directly over the heart. The electrodes irritated the skin and the patients found the repeated electric shocks painful.

After a power outage in 1957, Dr. C. Walton Lillehei (Figure 6), a pioneer in the nascent practice of open-heart surgery at the University of Minnesota in Minneapolis, MN, asked a local electrical engineer named Earl Bakken (Figure 7) to come up with a compact, lightweight, battery-operated pacing device.

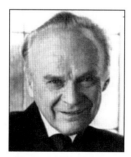 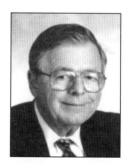

Figure 6. Dr. Walton Lillehei   **Figure 7.** Earl Bakken

A few weeks later Bakken brought Dr. Lillehei the world's first transistorized, battery-powered, wearable pacemaker (Figure 8). The device was powered by transistors and was equipped with myocardial leads that eliminated the old discomfort of electrodes attached to the skin. The device was soon in wide use for postoperative heart block following cardiac surgery.

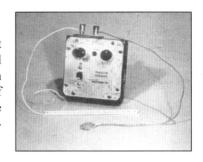

Figure 8. Medtronic first pacemaker built in 1957 by Earl Bakken for use by Dr. C. Walton Lillehei of the University of Minnesota Hospital. It was the world's first transistorized, battery-powered, wearable pacemaker.

Pacing technology had taken a giant step forward during the early and mid-1950s. It was however apparent that for long-term pacing a totally implanted device would have to be designed as ascending infection via the pacing electrodes occurred frequently (Figure 9). Dr. Lillehei himself noted: "The question of how long stimulation can be maintained appears to be related to electrode materials, design and technique of implantation…"

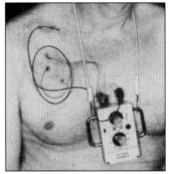

Figure 9. Wearable pacemaker with heart wires.

The availability of the semiconductor transistor, the development of biocompatible materials, and the refinement of open-heart surgery techniques made the next step (the fully implantable cardiac pacemaker), not only possible, but probably inevitable. In 1958, a Swedish team led by Dr. Åke Senning (Figure 10), and Rune Elmqvist (Figure 11), an engineer, implanted (in a heart-block patient) the first internal pacemaker (Figure 12).

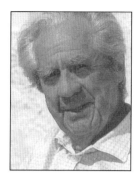 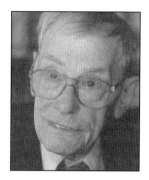

Figure 10. Dr. Åke Senning   **Figure 11.** Rune Elmqvist

Figure 12. Replica of the first implanted pacemaker. The entire unit was encapsulated in epoxy resin. Its diameter was approx. 55 mm, and it was 16 mm thick. The first units had two polyethylene-coated twisted stainless suture thread electrodes. The ends of these were fixed to the heart, and served as electrodes.

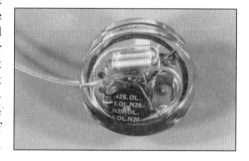

That device, incorporating a transistor and powered by a nickel-cadmium battery, functioned for three hours before failing; a second unit stimulated the patient for 8 days. Arne Larsson (the patient) survived both the engineer as well as the surgeon who had saved his life. He required five lead systems and 22 pulse generators of 11 different models until his death in 2001.

Also in 1958, Dr. William Chardack, Dr. Andrew Gage and electrical engineer Wilson Greatbatch (Figure 13) built, in Buffalo, NY, the first American implantable pacemaker. The three men carried out more than two years of experimental work and testing on animals. Finally, the Chardack-Greatbatch group reported its first human implantation in 1960.

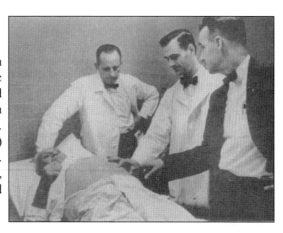

Figure 13. The implantation of the first cardiac pacemaker in the United States was performed on April 18, 1960, by Drs. William Chardack (left) and Andrew Gage (middle). Wilson Greatbatch (right), an engineer, designed and built the unit.

The Chardack-Greatbatch device incorporated yet another important component generated during the accelerating advance of pacing technology: the bipolar lead developed by St. Paul, MN, surgeon Dr. Samuel Hunter (Figure 14) and Medtronic engineer Norman Roth.

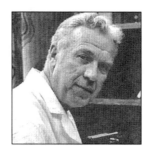

Figure 14. Dr. Samuel Hunter

The Hunter-Roth electrode, comprising a pair of stainless steel pins secured in a silicone rubber base (Figure 15), was implanted successfully in a 72-year-old Adams-Stokes disease patient in 1958 (Figure 16).

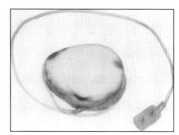

Figure 15. The Hunter-Roth bipolar lead (shown here with a Medtronic implantable pacemaker of 1960).

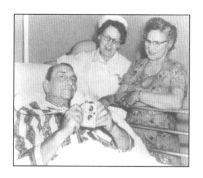

Figure 16. Warren Mauston, first recipient of the Hunter-Roth electrode, holds the battery-operated pulse generator developed by Earl Bakken in 1958. The patient recovered and lived an additional and active 7 years.

Other breakthroughs in lead technology were Chardack's invention of a myocardial electrode featuring a platinum/iridium spring coil and Dr. Seymour Furman's development of a transvenous insertion technique. Along with two colleagues, Dr. Furman (Figure 17) made history on July 16, 1958, at Montefiore Medical Center in the Bronx, NY, when he threaded plastic-coated wires connected to an electrode through the veins of a patient's heart, eliminating the need to cut the chest open (Figure 18).

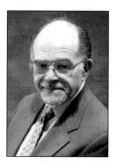

Figure 17. Dr. Seymour Furman

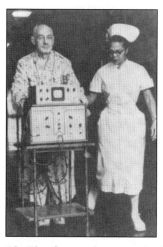

Figure 18. The first patient paced with a long-term transvenous lead, which was developed by Dr. Seymour Furman. Pacing was maintained for 96 days.

The endocardial lead was not welcomed enthusiastically in its early years of development. It was difficult to develop an unbreakable wire lead with an electrode that would remain in a stable position for a long period of time. Early adopters also reported myocardial perforation and high stimulation thresholds. As these problems were solved, the system gained wider acceptance among physicians; particularly since the transvenous lead could be implanted without a thoracotomy or general anesthesia.

Over the following decades, more durable, biocompatible materials for both the pulse generator and the leads have allowed manufacturers to overcome other problems such as: moisture damage, component fracture, and tissue reaction.

Cardiac defibrillation

The first instance of bizarre unregulated actions of the ventricles (later called ventricular fibrillation -VF) were produced, recorded and documented in 1850 by Carl Ludwig (Figure 19). Experiments were conducted by application of strong electrical current across animal hearts.

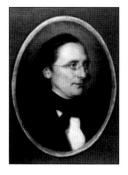

Figure 19. Carl Ludwig (German physician and professor of physiology).

In 1899, French physiologists, Jean Prevost (Figure 20) and Frédéric Battelli (Figure 21) were able to stop ventricular fibrillation (VF) in an animal by applying an electric shock to the exposed heart. They are credited for the first documented measurement of electrical current at various intensities and how it affected the electrical activity of animal hearts. Their work demonstrated that alternating current applied to the heart produced VF, and higher intensity terminated it.

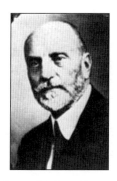 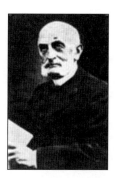

Figure 20. Jean Prevost   **Figure 21.** Frédéric Battelli

Prevost and Battelli's efforts went largely unnoticed for many years. The need to understand their work occurred in response to an increasing number of electric shock accidents and deaths. In 1930, an electricity company hired William Kouwenhoven (Figure 22), who reproduced with his colleagues the work of Prevost and Battelli and found that electrical current could cause VF, while an increase in that current could terminate it. The group of researchers also developed a closed-chest defibrillator that sent alternating current (AC) electrical shocks to an animal heart through electrodes placed on the chest.

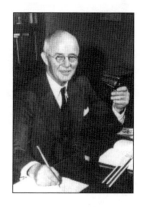

Figure 22. William Kouwenhoven, electrical engineer at Johns Hopkins University.

In 1947, the first successful human defibrillation was achieved by Claude Beck (Figure 23) and his colleagues. The cardiac arrest had occurred during surgery and electrical defibrillation was achieved at the second attempt by paddles (Figure 24) placed directly on the heart.

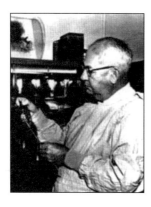

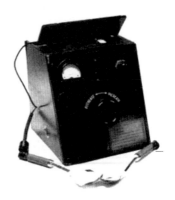

Figure 23. Dr. Claude Beck

Figure 24. The defibrillator with silver paddles (the size of large tablespoons) that were used in open-chest situations.

Dr. Paul Zoll is credited for the first human transthoracic defibrillation in 1956 (it was done with 7.5 cm diameter copper electrodes).

In 1970, Dr. Mieczyslaw Mirowski (Figure 25), a pioneered cardiologist, invented and co-developed an implantable device called the automatic implantable cardioverter defibrillator (AICD). The system used intracardiac catheter and patch electrodes (Figure 26).

Mirowski and co-workers implanted the first AICD in 1980 after a decade of research and animal experimentation.

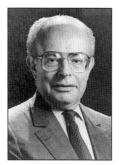

Figure 25. Dr. Mieczyslaw Mirowski

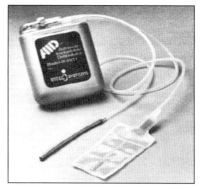

Figure 26. The first human grade automatic implantable cardioverter defibrillator with a patch and catheter electrode.

The AICD implantation methods evolved as technology progressed. The large devices of the 1980s were implanted in the abdomen with epicardial patch leads tunneled down to the abdomen. Then, as lead technology advanced to allow for venous approach, the leads were tunneled down from the subclavian area to the abdomen. Today, the small size of an ICD allows for device implantation in the pectoral area with a transvenous lead system.

CHAPTER 2

Cardiovascular System, Cardiac Rhythm and Disorders

Heart

The cardiac muscle is shaped to form four cardiac chambers. Each of the two upper chambers is called an atrium, and each lower chamber is called a ventricle. Each chamber of the heart has its own function. As simplified in Figure 1, the right atrium receives the "used up" blood from all parts of the body. This blood is depleted of oxygen but contains high levels of carbon dioxide from metabolism in the body's tissues. The right atrium contracts and pumps this blood through the tricuspid valve into the right ventricle. The blood is then pumped from the right ventricle through the pulmonary valve into the pulmonary artery, which delivers the blood to the lungs. In the lungs the blood takes on oxygen and gives-up its carbon dioxide. During normal breathing carbon dioxide is expelled from the lungs while oxygen is taken in. The newly oxygenated blood travels from the lungs through the pulmonary veins to the left atrium. The oxygenated blood is pumped from the left atrium, through the mitral valve, into the left ventricle. The left ventricle is the more important of the two lower chambers, and it is supplied with blood through three coronary arteries. Finally, during contraction of the left ventricle, the oxygen-rich blood is pumped through the aortic valve into the aorta and branching arteries to be delivered to all the organs of the body, including the brain, heart, kidneys, and muscles. The body tissues utilize the oxygen for fuel and deliver the waste carbon dioxide back to the blood, which returns to the right atrium through veins, and the cycle continues.

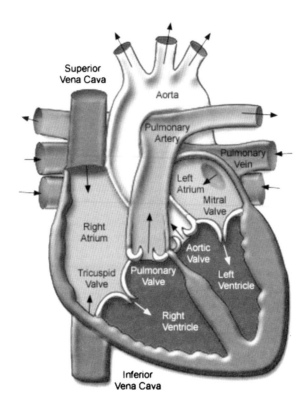

Figure 1. Illustration of blood flow through the heart.

Electrical conduction system

During a normal human's lifetime, the heart beats an estimated three billion times. Each beat is coordinated by a sophisticated network of neural tissue known as the cardiac conduction system or CCS. The CCS generates electrical impulses which are rapidly conducted through the heart muscle. This impulse causes the heart chambers to contract in a rhythmic sequence, pumping blood throughout the body.

As described in Figure 2, the elements comprising the CCS are the sinoatrial node ("SA node" or "natural pacemaker"), the atrioventricular node ("AV node"), the bundle of His, the right and left branches and the Purkinje fibers.

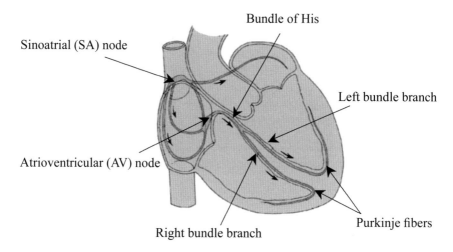

Figure 2. Representation of the electrical conduction system.

The SA node is a small lump of neural tissue located in the right atrium of the heart. This tiny cluster of cells is responsible for initiating the electrical impulse that causes the heart to beat. This impulse travels rapidly throughout the cells of the atria causing them to contract then continues on to the AV node. Located near the center of the heart, the AV node serves as a "gatekeeper" delaying the electrical impulse before relaying it on to stimulate the ventricles. This slight delay ensures that the right and left atria have had sufficient time to contract before the ventricles do. From here, the impulse travels on to the right and left ventricles by way of the bundle of His, the right and left bundle branches and the conduction pathways. These specialized nerve fibers are located inside the muscular walls of the heart. The impulse is passed through the muscle cells of the ventricles causing them to contract and forcefully eject the blood contained within.

Heart beat anatomy

After the SA node fires, the resulting depolarization wave passes through the right and left atria, which produces the P-wave on the electrocardiogram (ECG/EKG) surface and stimulates the atrial contraction (Figure 3).

Following activation of the atria, the impulse proceeds to the atrioventricular (AV) node, which is the only normal conduction pathway between the atria and the ventricles. The AV node slows impulse conduction, which allows time for the atria to contract and for blood to be pumped from the atria to the ventricles prior to ventricular contraction. Conduction time through the AV node accounts for most of the duration of the PR interval. Just below the AV node, the impulse passes through the bundle of His. A small portion of the last part of the PR interval is represented by the conduction time through the bundle of His.

The impulse passes quickly through the bundle of His, the left and right bundle branches, and the Purkinje fibers, leading to depolarization and contraction of the ventricles. The QRS complex on the EKG represents the depolarization of the ventricular muscle mass. Repolarization of the ventricles generates a current in the body fluids and produces a T-wave. This takes place slowly, and generates a wide wave.

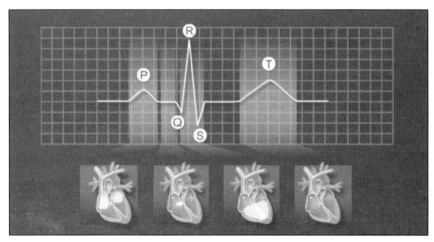

Figure 3. EKG wave represented with respect to the heart function associated with it.

Heart rhythm disorders

The heart's electrical system can be affected in many ways by disease. The SA node, the AV node, or other areas of the electrical system can malfunction and trigger arrhythmias (Figures 4 thru 8).

Cardiovascular System, Cardiac Rhythm and Disorders 17

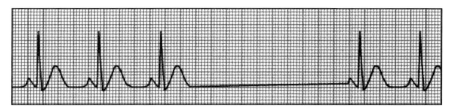

Figure 4. Sinus arrest (pause in the rate at which the SA node fires).

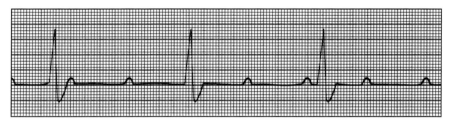

Figure 5. Complete AV block (also referred to as complete heart block). It is characterized by a complete dissociation between P-waves and QRS complexes.

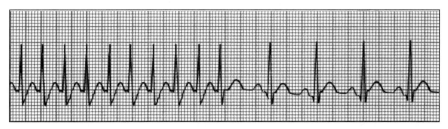

Figure 6. Paroxysmal atrial tachycardia. Periods of very rapid and regular heart beats that begins and ends abruptly (the term paroxysmal means that the event begins suddenly, without warning, and ends abruptly). The EKG deflection shows a rapid heart rate (range between 160-200 BPM) a normal P and R-wave depolarization.

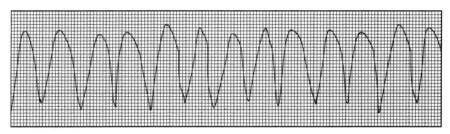

Figure 7. Ventricular tachycardia (VT). The EKG deflection shows rapid (>150 BPM), wide and bizarre QRS complexes. Ventricular tachycardia can quickly deteriorate into ventricular fibrillation.

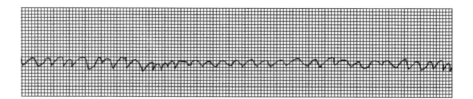

Figure 8. Ventricular fibrillation (VF). The EKG deflection shows a heart rhythm highly irregular (P-waves and QRS complexes are not present).

A disruption in impulse formation and/or conduction can result in abnormal heartbeats from very slow heart rates (bradycardias) to very fast heart rates (tachycardias). Implantable pacemakers and leads are most often used to treat severe bradycardia from abnormal SA node function or impaired or absent conduction through the AV node.

Two common life-threatening tachycardias are ventricular tachycardia (VT) and ventricular fibrillation (VF). VT is a rapid regular rhythm caused by electrical signals originating from an area of the ventricle. VT can decrease blood delivery by the heart and cause low blood pressure and can also progress to a more serious heart rhythm called VF. VF is an irregular rhythm, which is a result of multiple rapid and chaotic electrical signals firing from many different areas in the ventricles. A heart undergoing VF is in a state of standstill called cardiac arrest. The heart muscles quiver and cease pumping which causes a halt in the delivery of blood to the body. Unless VF is terminated quickly, irreversible brain damage occurs within minutes of the onset of ventricular fibrillation, leading to death. Implantable cardioverter defibrillators (ICD) and leads deliver electrical impulses and high energy discharges to treat tachycardias (they also provide bradycardia pacing when needed).

Heart failure

Heart failure (HF) is a condition that reduces the heart's ability to pump blood. It can result from a heart attack, untreated high blood pressure, or an abnormality of one of the heart valves. Because of HF, the damaged muscle is a less effective pump resulting in a reduced ability to supply oxygen to meet the needs of the body and brain.

In the normal heart, the ventricles pump at the same time and in synchronization with the atria. When the contractions become out of synchronization, the left ventricle is not able to pump enough blood to the body. This eventually leads to an increase in HF symptoms, such as shortness of breath, dry cough, swelling in the ankles or legs, weight gain, increased urination, fatigue, or rapid or irregular heartbeat.

The New York Heart Association (NYHA) functional classification provides a simple way of classifying the extent of HF. It places patients in one of four categories (Table 1) based on how much they are limited during physical activity.

Table 1 – NYHA Class

NYHA Class	Extent of HF
I	No symptoms and no limitation in ordinary physical activity.
II	Mild symptoms (mild shortness of breath and/or angina pain) and slight limitation during ordinary activity.
III	Marked limitation in activity due to symptoms, even during less-than-ordinary activity (e.g. walking short distances). Comfortable only at rest.
IV	Severe limitations. Experiences symptoms even while at rest.

Ejection fraction (EF) is one of the measurements used by physicians to assess how well a patient's heart is functioning. "Ejection" refers to the amount of blood that is pumped out of the heart's main pumping chamber during each heartbeat. "Fraction" refers to the fact that, even in a healthy heart, some blood always remains within this chamber after each heartbeat. Therefore an EF is a percentage of the blood within the chamber that is pumped out with every heartbeat. An EF of 55 to 75 percent is considered normal. A low EF could be a sign that the heart is weakened.

Conventional pacemakers are used to regulate the heart rate and keep the atrium and ventricle working together (this is called AV synchrony). Cardiac resynchronization therapy (CRT) devices (also known as biventricular pacemakers) are implanted in patients with symptoms of severe HF, systolic left ventricular dysfunction, and ventricular dysynchrony. They are designed to treat the delay in the ventricle contractions by keeping the right and left ventricles pumping together (Figure 9 illustrates 3 levels of coordinated electromechanical synchrony that are relevant to the implementation of CRT with pacing). As a result of improved synchrony, systole becomes more effective and therefore EF, cardiac output (CO), and other parameters of cardiac function are improved.

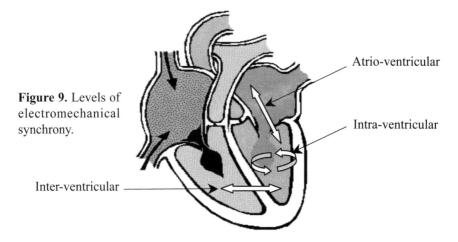

Figure 9. Levels of electromechanical synchrony.

CRT by means of biventricular pacing is a fairly new procedure that was approved by the United States Food and Drug Administration (FDA) in 2001. Many studies that have been published suggest that CRT improves patient quality of life (based on the Minnesota

Living with Heart Failure Quality of Life Questionnaire), increases distance walked in 6 minutes, improves oxygen uptake, lowers NYHA classification, decreases QRS duration, increases left ventricular EF, and increases peak oxygen consumption.

In standard biventricular pacing, leads are implanted into the right atrium, the right ventricle and into the coronary sinus vein (Figure 10) to pace or regulate the left ventricle. The combination of all three leads creates a synchronized pumping of the ventricles, increasing the efficiency of each beat and pumping more blood on the whole.

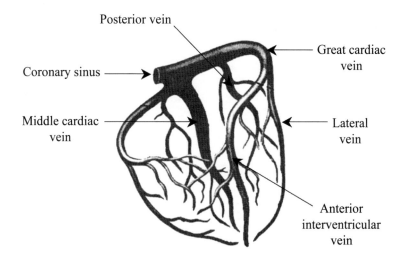

Figure 10. Cardiac venous anatomy.

CHAPTER 3

Pacing Lead Terminology and Technology

Description of an implantable pacing system

In general, pacing systems are used to control a patient's heart rate when the intrinsic rate is inappropriate for the patient's needs. A system consists of an implantable pulse generator (IPG) and one or two leads (Figure 1). The IPG contains the battery and various circuits that control pacemaker operations. Most IPGs have a telemetry coil for sending programming instructions and receiving diagnostic data. Many have sensors that measure indicators of exertion and use the results to change heart rate.

Brady leads are insulated conductor wires that deliver electrical impulses to the heart and return sensed electrical signals from the heart to the IPG. One end of the lead connects to the IPG and the other is in contact with the cardiac tissue.

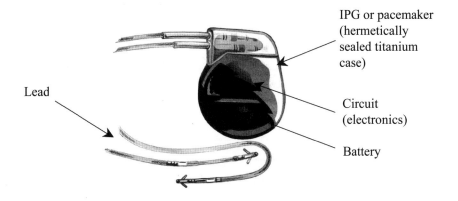

Figure 1. Illustration of a pacing system.

Construction and components

The main components of passive fixation leads are shown below:

Unipolar straight passive fixation lead

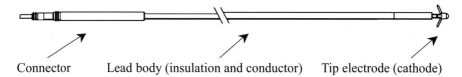

Bipolar straight passive fixation lead

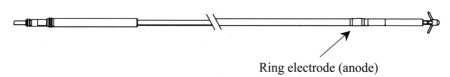

Bipolar "J" shape passive fixation lead

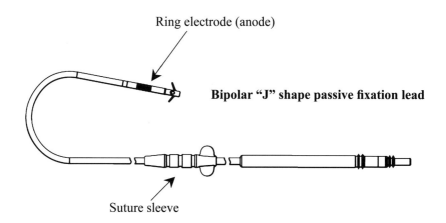

Passive fixation means that no part of the lead itself is actually embedded in the endocardium; rather, the lead tip is trapped within the trabeculae (Figure 2) and/or is held in position by its pre-formed shape.

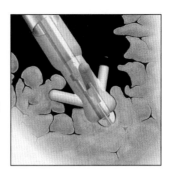

Figure 2. Passive fixation lead tip trapped in trabeculae.

Straight leads are usually implanted in the apex of the right ventricle and "J" leads are pre-shaped for positioning in the right atrial appendage (Figure 3).

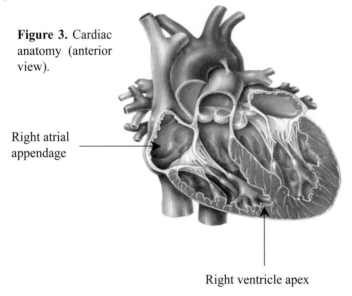

Figure 3. Cardiac anatomy (anterior view).

Right atrial appendage

Right ventricle apex

The main components of active fixation leads are shown below:

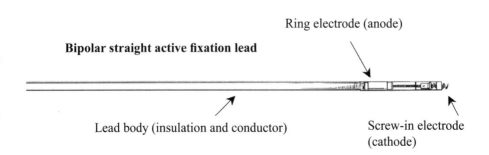

Bipolar straight active fixation lead

Ring electrode (anode)

Lead body (insulation and conductor)

Screw-in electrode (cathode)

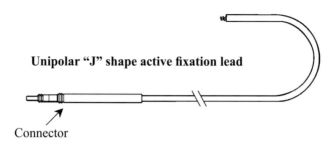

Active fixation means that part of the lead actually embeds in the heart tissue for fixation, for example a screw-in helix electrode (Figure 4).

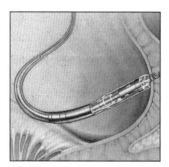

Figure 4. Screw-in helix electrode embedded in heart tissue.

Polarity

Both unipolar and bipolar pacing leads require a tip electrode (cathode) and an indifferent electrode (anode) to complete the electrical circuit. In unipolar construction, the conductor carries the pacing stimulus to the tip electrode that is in contact with the myocardium. The primary construction difference between unipolar and bipolar leads is in the location of the indifferent electrode. In unipolar pacing, cardiac tissue, body tissue and body fluid carry the electrical current back to the indifferent electrode which is the pulse generator case. In bipolar pacing, a second conductor carries electrical current back from the indifferent electrode or ring electrode to the pulse generator.

A unipolar lead has one conductor wire and one electrode at the tip of the lead body. The cathode is in contact with the heart and the anode is the IPG can.

In a unipolar system, a pacing pulse travels from the IPG to the tip electrode (cathode) to stimulate the heart; then it returns to the IPG can through the chest tissues to complete the pacing circuit as illustrated in Figure 5.

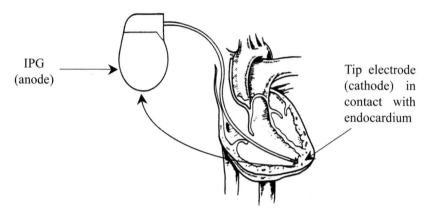

Figure 5. Current flows through a substantial part of the chest and form a large current loop.

A bipolar lead has two conductor wires and both anode and cathode are in the heart (Figure 6). In a bipolar system, a pacing pulse travels from the IPG to the tip electrode and then to the ring electrode. It returns to the IPG by way of a second conductor wire.

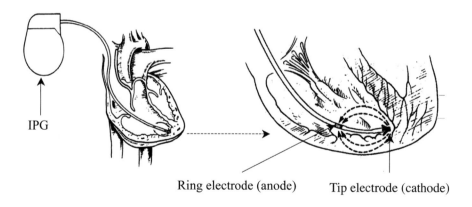

Figure 6. Illustration of a bipolar lead configuration. The anode is the ring electrode located 1 to 2 cm (the distance varies with manufacturer and lead design) above the cathode.

The advantages and disadvantages of unipolar and bipolar stimulations are illustrated in Figure 7 and summarized below:
- Inappropriate stimulation is sometimes an effect of unipolar pacing configurations (this happens when an electric impulse returning to the pacemaker stimulates muscles near it, most commonly the pectoral muscles).
- Lead size is important in leads that are threaded transvenously. Unipolar leads are less rigid (there is only one conductor coil and one layer of insulation). Bipolar leads were once much larger than they are today so size is becoming less of an issue between unipolar and bipolar systems.

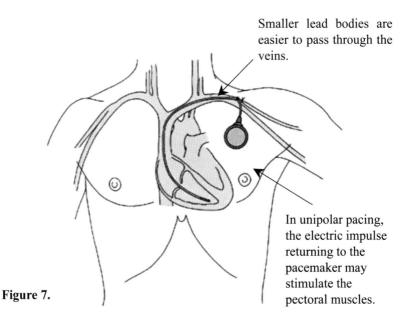

Figure 7.

Smaller lead bodies are easier to pass through the veins.

In unipolar pacing, the electric impulse returning to the pacemaker may stimulate the pectoral muscles.

- Redundancy is built into a bipolar system because if a lead conductor fractures, the system can be converted to a unipolar lead system through pacemaker programming. The unipolar system only has one conductor and has no similar back-up.
- Programming flexibility is built into a bipolar lead because they can be programmed to either unipolar or bipolar configurations.

- Sensing in bipolar systems is somewhat superior to that of unipolar systems. Bipolar leads can sense cardiac depolarization more accurately. They are also less likely to sense electrical signals from outside the heart, such as from other muscles or from electromagnetic interference.
- Unipolar signals are larger than bipolar ones.

Length and diameter

Leads are available in a wide array of lengths (40 to 80 cm). Shorter and longer units can be manufactured to give physicians additional treatment options and to accommodate specific patient needs.

The French catheter scale is commonly used to measure the outside diameter of cylindrical medical instruments including leads. The "French Gauge", as it is also known, was invented by Joseph-Frédéric-Benoît Charrière (Figure 8), a 19th century Parisian maker of surgical instruments, who defined the "diameter times 3" relationship.

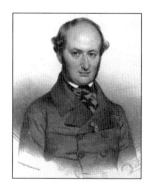

Figure 8. Joseph-Frédéric-Benoît Charrière developed a standard gauge specifically designed for use in medical equipment such as catheters and probes. This system is commonly referred to as French (Fr) sizing.

In the French system, the diameter in millimeters can be determined by dividing the French size by 3, thus an increasing French size corresponds with a larger diameter catheter. The following equations summarize the relationships:

$$D \text{ (mm)} = F/3 \text{ or } F = D \text{ (mm)} * 3$$

For example, if the French size of a lead is 9, the diameter is 3 mm (Table 1).

Table 1.

French Gauge	Diameter (mm)	Diameter (inches)
1	0,33	0.013
2	0,66	0.026
3	1	0.039
4	1,35	0.053
5	1,67	0.066
6	2	0.079
7	2,3	0.092
8	2,7	0.105
9	3	0.118

CHAPTER 4

Tachy Lead Terminology and Technology

Description of an implantable cardioverter defibrillator system

A defibrillation system consists of an implantable cardioverter defibrillator (also called defibrillator or ICD) and one or more leads. The defibrillator unit is a small titanium case containing electronic circuits, capacitor(s), and battery (Figure 1). The leads help the defibrillator unit monitor the natural heart rhythm and deliver electrical shock(s) from the ICD to the heart when tachycardia occurs. The microchip runs the defibrillator, monitors the heart rhythm, instructs the capacitor(s) to send electrical shock(s) when tachycardia occurs, determines the strength of the shock(s) sent, and also keeps a record of the heart rhythms as well as the shock(s) sent by the defibrillator.

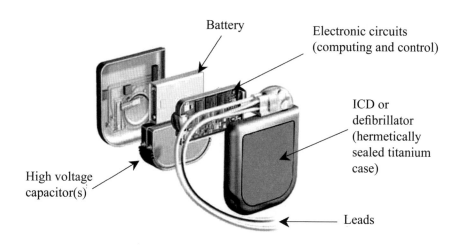

Figure 1. Illustration of a defibrillation system.

32 Chapter 4

Specialized electronic circuits in the ICD have voltage multiplying capabilities. They can produce up to 800 Volts for storage of a large amount of energy (30 to 35 joules) in the capacitors. This energy is delivered to the heart at a precise time when a shock is needed.

The ICD identifies abnormal heart rhythms and determines the appropriate therapy to return a patient's heartbeat to a normal heart rhythm. The therapies are programmed to ensure maximum patient safety while attempting to deliver the less aggressive treatment (less painful and least impact on device longevity) that will terminate the arrhythmia. The ICD therapies can be tiered; such that the device initially delivers less aggressive treatments that are subsequently increased in aggressiveness until the desired treatment is obtained. The physician can program the ICD to include one or all of the following functions:

- <u>Bradycardia pacing</u> – When the heart beats too slow, small electrical impulses are sent to stimulate the heart muscle.
- <u>Anti-tachycardia pacing (ATP)</u> – When the heart beats too fast, a series of small electrical impulses are delivered to the heart muscle to restore a normal heart rate and rhythm (Figure 2).
- <u>Cardioversion therapy</u> – A low energy shock is delivered at the same time as the heartbeat (synchronized shock on R wave) to restore a normal heart rhythm.
- <u>Defibrillation therapy</u> – When the heart is beating dangerously fast, a high energy shock (asynchronous) is delivered to the heart muscle to restore a normal rhythm (Figure 3).

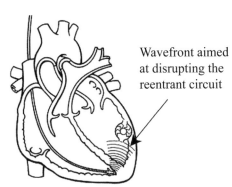

Wavefront aimed at disrupting the reentrant circuit

Figure 2. Low voltage pulses delivered to a small cluster of cells.

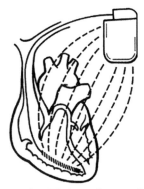

Figure 3. High voltage shock delivered over a mass of cells.

Evolution of technology

Figure 4 exhibits the impressive reduction in size of ICDs from 1989 to 1996. Simultaneous improvements were made in battery longevity, efficacy, diagnostics and memory capabilities.

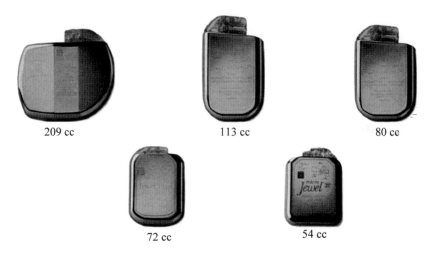

Figure 4. Medtronic first ICD (1989) had a volume of 209 cc and lasted about two years (the device was called a pacemaker cardioverter defibrillator or PCD, and required abdominal implant because of its size and weight). Today, single and dual-chamber units are about 35 cc (reduction in size and weight allows for pectoral implant) with a six to seven-year longevity, depending on how often they discharge.

Research on implantable defibrillators was initiated in the early 1970s. The emergence of advanced technologies in circuit miniaturization, battery and circuit composition led to the development of devices designed to control occurrences of ventricular arrhythmias. In the late 1980s, the PCD was the first device on the market capable of offering a range of automatically administered therapies (tiered therapy) for controlling potentially life-threatening occurrences of ventricular arrhythmias. If a patient experienced ventricular tachycardia (VT), the PCD was able to restore a normal rhythm by pacing before triggering more aggressive treatments of cardioversion or defibrillation. When first introduced, the PCD used epicardial patch leads. These leads required that the patient's chest be opened so that the patches could be attached to the surface of the heart (Figures 5 and 6).

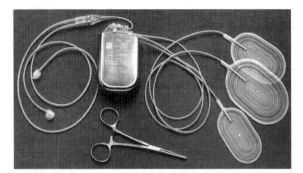 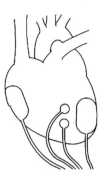

Figure 5. PCD with 3 patch leads. The 2 smaller electrodes shown on the left are the pacing electrodes adapted as a bifurcated bipolar system.

Figure 6. Illustration of a two-patch system. The PCD is implanted in the abdomen. One patch on the posterolateral left ventricle, the second patch on the anterior right ventricle and the myocardial pace/sense electrodes toward the ventricular apex.

Epicardial patch leads were placed directly on the epicardium of the heart and sutured for fixation. They had several oval shaped coils of wire designed for flexibility (Figure 7). The platinum alloy coils were imbedded in a flexible silicone pad, which allowed the patch to flex with contractions of the heart.

Figure 7. Sutures are placed through the outer skirt of the patch. The flexible silicone pad allows the patch to flex with contractions of the heart.

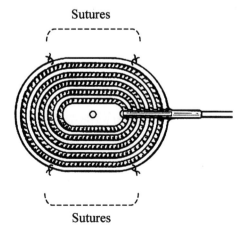

Epicardial patches should not be confused with subcutaneous patches (SQ patch) which are implanted under the skin, not on the epicardium of the heart. They were stiffer and used occasionally as an added electrode to a transvenous lead system (Figure 8). Also, as lead technology advanced to allow for venous approach, the leads were tunneled down from the subclavian area to the abdomen where a pocket was created for the device.

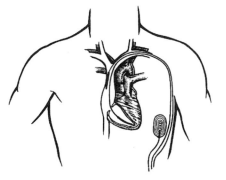

Figure 8. Transvenous and SQ patch leads with an abdominal ICD placement (device not shown).

Today, the small size of an ICD allows for device implantation in the pectoral area with a transvenous lead system (Figure 9).

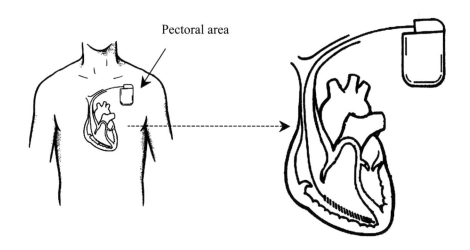

Figure 9. ICD implanted in the pectoral area with a transvenous lead.

Construction and components

Tachy leads (also known as tachycardia leads, high-voltage leads or defibrillation leads) are leads through which an ICD delivers shocks. They are referred to as transvenous leads and are categorized according to their method of fixation:

- Active fixation means that part of the lead actually embeds in the heart tissue via a screw-in helix electrode (Figure 10).

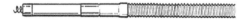

Figure 10. Active fixation design (helix electrode extended).

- Passive fixation (Figure 11) allows the tip of the lead to anchor itself into a stable position (the tip is trapped within the trabeculae).

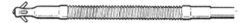

Figure 11. Passive fixation design.

- No Fixation (Figure 12) high voltage leads serve generally as an added high voltage coil electrode. The coil ends up "floating" inside the superior vena cava or in the coronary sinus.

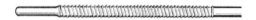

Figure 12. No fixation concept.

Except for the standardized connectors, the construction of the lead bodies, conductors, and electrodes vary among manufacturers. Figures 13 and 14 illustrate the construction of a single coil active fixation and a dual coil passive fixation leads respectively.

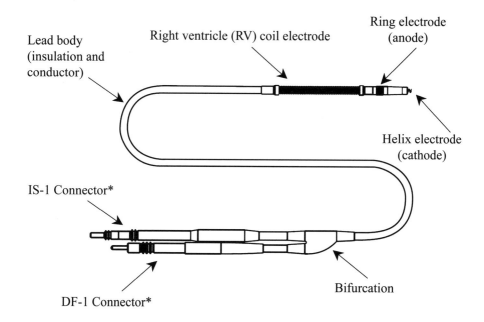

Figure 13. Single coil active fixation lead (tripolar).

* Earlier ICDs and tachy leads had various styles of connectors for mating leads to the devices. Adapters had to be designed for connecting leads to different models of ICDs. Eventually, device manufacturers agreed upon international standards for a basic mechanical fit of lead connectors into device connector blocks. The pace/sense connections use the IS-1 International Connector Standard for pacemakers. For the high-voltage connections, an International Connector Standard (ISO 11318) was developed and identified as DF-1.

The three electrodes of the lead are the helix, the ring, and the RV coil.
- The helix electrode is common to the connector pin of the IS-1 bipolar connector.
- The ring electrode is common to the connector ring of the IS-1 bipolar connector.
- The RV coil electrode is common to the connector pin of the DF-1 unipolar connector.

The IS-1 bipolar leg of the bifurcation features a lumen for stylet passage. The DF-1 connector does not accept a stylet. The RV coil delivers cardioversion and defibrillation therapies. Pacing and sensing occur between the helix and ring electrodes. While sharing similarities with other leads, the tachy leads also have to transmit high voltage shocks (up to 800 Volts) from the device to the heart. The energy is transmitted via special components and dedicated circuits with low resistance to maximize defibrillation of the heart cells. The conductors are cables (drawn brazed strand or MP35N composite).

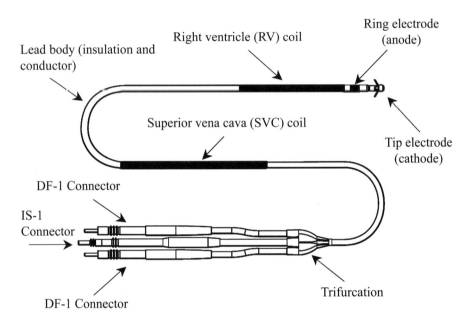

Figure 14. Dual coil passive fixation lead (quadripolar).

The four electrodes of the lead are the tip, the ring, the RV and SVC coils.
- The tip electrode is common to the connector pin of the IS-1 bipolar leg.
- The ring electrode is common to the connector ring of the IS-1 bipolar leg.
- The RV electrode coil is common to the DF-1 RV leg of the trifurcation.
- The SVC electrode coil is common to the DF-1 SVC leg of the trifurcation.

The IS-1 bipolar leg of the trifurcation features a lumen for stylet passage. The DF-1 connectors will not accept a stylet. The RV and SVC coils deliver cardioversion and defibrillation therapies. Pacing and sensing occur between the tip and ring electrodes.

SVC/CS defib leads have no fixation mechanism (Figure 15). SVC lead design lets the coil electrode "floats" inside the superior vena cava while CS design allows the coil electrode to be positioned inside the coronary sinus. Both designs generally serve as an added circuit to maximize defibrillation thresholds.

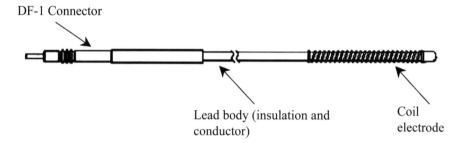

Figure 15. Superior vena cava/coronary sinus (SVC/CS) lead (unipolar).

Historically, patients with higher energy delivery requirements would receive a patch electrode implanted under the skin (with all the complications and discomfort associated with it). The SQ lead (Figure 16) is intended for use if a standard ICD system with one or two transvenous leads has not been efficacious in providing acceptable defibrillation threshold (DFT) measurements.

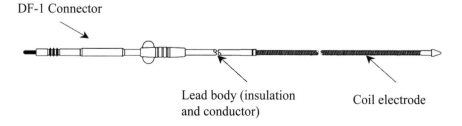

Figure 16. Subcutaneous (SQ) lead (unipolar).

The SQ lead provides an easier and less invasive implantation method (Figure 17).

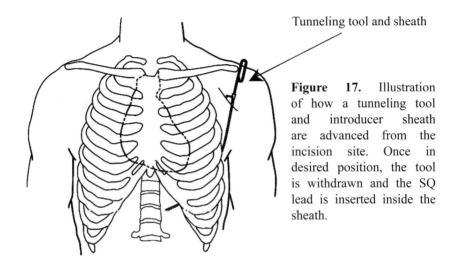

Figure 17. Illustration of how a tunneling tool and introducer sheath are advanced from the incision site. Once in desired position, the tool is withdrawn and the SQ lead is inserted inside the sheath.

Another subcutaneous lead design consists of 3 electrically common coils that form one electrode (Figure 18). The coils come together in an insulated cable that is connected to a connector pin. The "array" provides a greater surface area to maximize the defibrillation success.

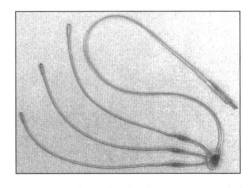

Figure 18. Subcutaneous array lead (courtesy of Boston Scientific).

High voltage transvenous leads can be single lumen, coaxial or multilumen. A single lumen design has a central conductor surrounded by insulation (Figure 19). A coaxial construction has conductors embedded within concentric layers of insulation (Figure 20). Multilumen design (Figure 21) allows having smaller diameter leads able to perform similar functions.

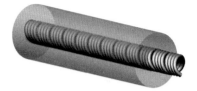

Figure 19. Single lumen lead design.

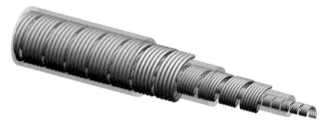

Figure 20. Coaxial construction (lead body diameter tends to be high for the multiple layers of insulation, body stiffness is also substantial).

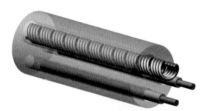

Figure 21. Multilumen design (extruded polymer insulates the conductors from one another).

Polarity

In a true bipolar configuration, the impulse flows through the tip electrode (cathode) located at the end of the lead, stimulates the heart, and returns to the ring electrode (anode). An ICD lead may sometimes use the high voltage RV coil to serve as the anode electrode to complete a bipolar circuit. This type of lead is known as an integrated bipolar lead because the anode is integrated into the high voltage coil (Figures 22 and 23 illustrates the concept for active and passive fixation leads).

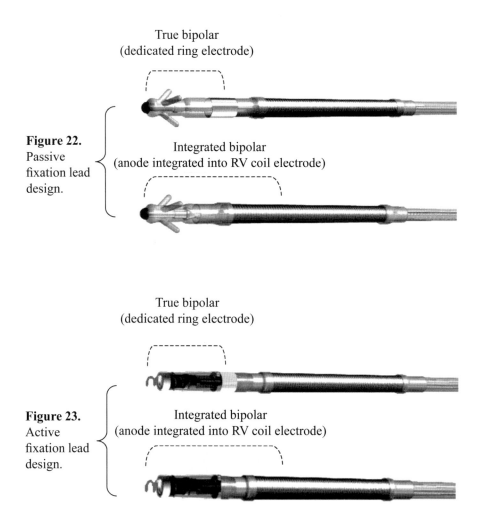

Figure 22. Passive fixation lead design.

Figure 23. Active fixation lead design.

Shocking circuits

A shocking circuit (also known as shocking vector) describes the high voltage pathway being used to deliver cardioversion or defibrillation therapy. If the HV lead has only one coil electrode, the pathway is between the device (acting as an active can) and the RV coil (Figure 24). The shaded area (Figure 25) illustrates the effect of the shock onto the mass of heart cells.

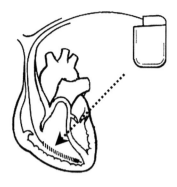 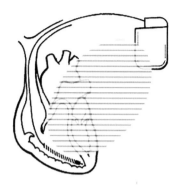

Figure 24. Shocking vector from device (active can) to RV coil electrode.

Figure 25. Electric field between ICD (acting as an electrode) and RV coil electrode.

When the HV lead is dual coil (RV and SVC coil electrodes), the pathways are between the ICD (active can) and the RV coil and between the SVC and RV coils (Figure 26). The shaded areas (Figure 27) illustrate the effect of the shock onto a larger mass of heart cells.

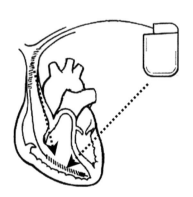 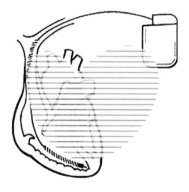

Figure 26. Shocking vectors from device (active can) to RV coil electrode and from SVC coil electrode to RV coil electrode.

Figure 27. Electric fields between ICD (acting as an electrode) and RV coil electrode and between SVC coil electrode and RV coil electrode.

Length (and surface area) of coil electrodes, lead placement, and device implant location play an important role in the delivery of the therapy.

When a lead has two coil electrodes (RV and SVC), the implanting physician has the option to disable the active can and to deliver the energy from coil to coil (Figure 28).

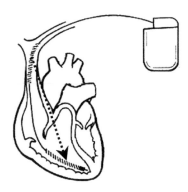

Figure 28. Shocking vector from SVC coil electrode to RV coil electrode.

Also, some devices allow the shocking vectors to be programmed to reverse the flow of energy and make the defibrillation more effective (Figures 29 and 30).

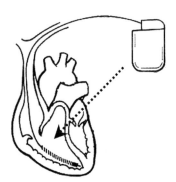 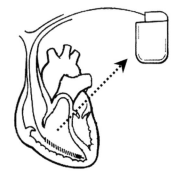

Figure 29. First therapy from device (active can) to RV coil electrode.

Figure 30. Second therapy from RV coil electrode to device.

Coil electrode

Electrical defibrillation electrodes utilize coil electrode construction. Coils offer efficient surface area over a broad and flexible region creating a large electric field (refer to Figures 31-33 for illustrations of energy distribution). Defibrillation coils have traditionally been made from platinum/iridium for biostability and biocompatibility. To improve electrical efficiency, low resistance core materials are now used within the wire.

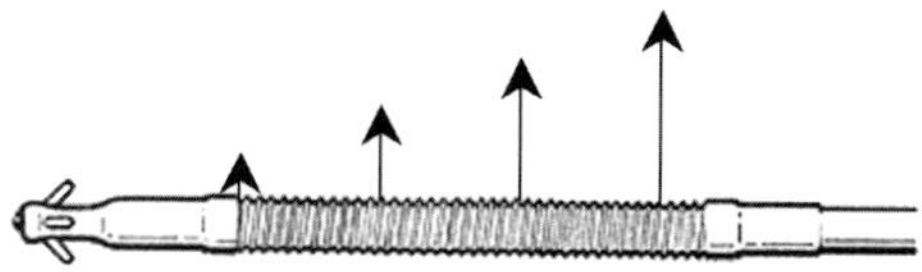

Figure 31. Coil electrode is connected proximally (the spread of energy decreases as it travels from the proximal connection).

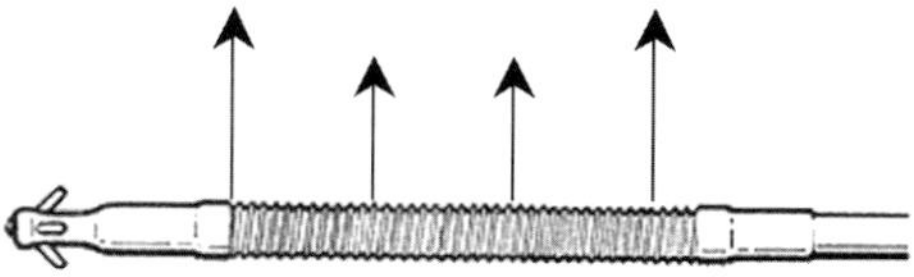

Figure 32. Coil electrode connected on both extremities (improved current distribution along the coil).

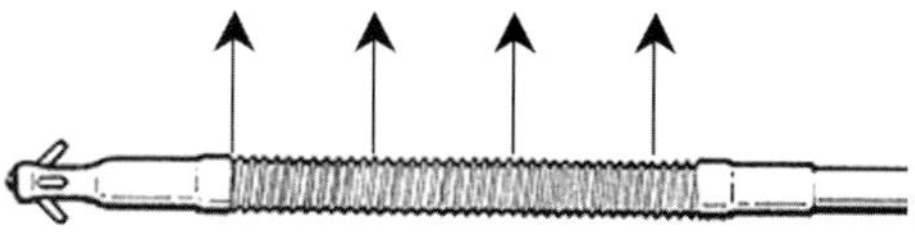

Figure 33. More uniform current distribution with dual connection and lower resistance coil electrode.

Transvenous leads adhere to the inner walls of the great veins, right atrium, and right ventricle over time. The coil electrodes provide a large surface area for scar ingrowth, and typically represent sites for significant binding (Figure 34), increasing the difficulty and risk of subsequent lead extraction, should that be needed for mechanical or infective complications.

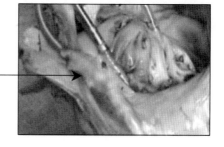

Figure 34. Fibrotic tissue around lead body and coil electrode.

Some lead designs incorporate sleeves of expanded polytetrafluoroethylene (ePTFE) GORE-TEX® that covers the coil electrodes (Figure 35), with the goal of preventing tissue in-growth between the coil filars and thereby improving the success and safety of future lead extraction.

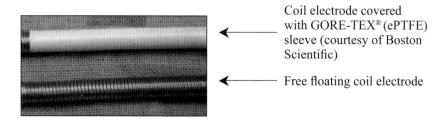

Coil electrode covered with GORE-TEX® (ePTFE) sleeve (courtesy of Boston Scientific)

Free floating coil electrode

Figure 35.

Silicone rubber backfill of the defibrillation coil is another alternative to prevent tissue in-growth between and around the coil wires (filars). With free floating coils on the lead body, encapsulation tissue can grow around the defibrillation electrode coil wire (see Figure 36 for illustration of concepts).

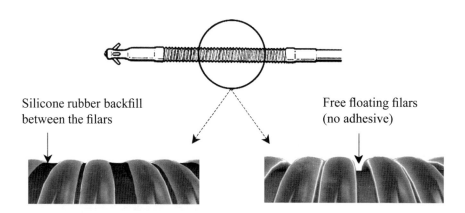

Silicone rubber backfill between the filars

Free floating filars (no adhesive)

Figure 36. Coil electrode construction.

CHAPTER 5

CRT Lead and Delivery System Terminology and Technology

Description of an implantable biventricular pacing system

A biventricular pacing system consists of an implantable pulse generator (IPG) and three leads (Figure 1). The system is also known as cardiac resynchronization therapy – pacing (CRT-P) for having the third lead to resynchronize the pumping action of the heart.

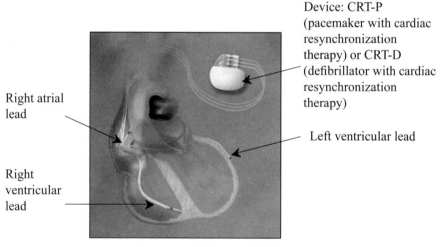

Figure 1. Illustration of a biventricular pacing system.

The resynchronization was initially accomplished by using a standard right ventricular lead and an epimyocardial lead which were connected with an adapter. It soon became apparent that it was undesirable to subject the patients to a thoracotomy for the placement of an epimyocardial lead, and entire transvenous systems were developed. Current biventricular pacing systems have leads that are placed in the right atrium and right ventricle. The left ventricular (LV) lead is placed via the coronary sinus in a cardiac vein, preferably a lateral or postero-lateral vein in the mid part of the LV (Figure 2).

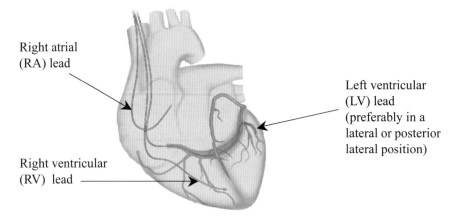

Figure 2. Typical lead placement for a biventricular pacing system.

Construction and components

The main components of LV leads (also known as CRT or left heart leads) are shown below:

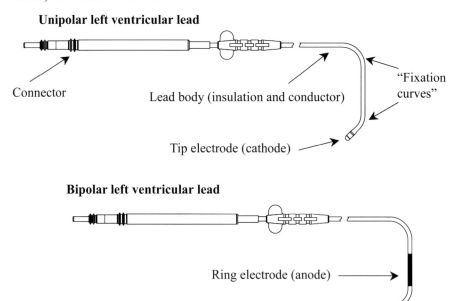

Characteristics of LV leads are quite similar to other leads:
- Polarity can either be unipolar or bipolar.
- Silicone and polyurethane are used as prime insulation.
- Conductor mostly made of MP35N.
- Electrodes (with or without steroid).
- Connectors (IS-1 unipolar or IS-1 bipolar).
- Suture sleeve to reduce possibility of CS lead dislodgement and to protect the lead insulation and conductor coil from damage caused by tight ligatures.

While sharing similarities with brady leads components and materials, they have distinctive shapes to allow CS cannulation and to provide a mean of fixation in the cardiac veins.

Delivery systems and fixation mechanisms

CRT leads are intended to pace the left side of the heart but they are not placed in the left ventricle. The leads are located inside the coronary sinus (CS) or in one of the cardiac veins. Although they pose unique challenges to the implanting physician, these locations have demonstrated stable implant sites and offer viable options to stimulate the outside of the left ventricle. Figure 3 shows an early lead design for placement in the CS (this lead generation was stylet delivered and had limited maneuverability to advance further down the veins).

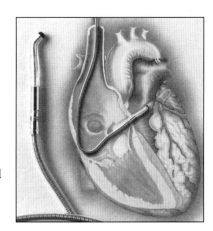

Figure 3. Stylet delivered LV lead.

Subsequently various implantation tools (also known as guiding catheters or sheaths) were made available to cannulate the CS (Figure 4) and to select a cardiac vein.

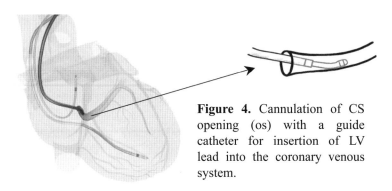

Figure 4. Cannulation of CS opening (os) with a guide catheter for insertion of LV lead into the coronary venous system.

Some systems offer preformed curves to accommodate patient's heart anatomy (Figures 5 and 6). Fixed shape catheters can have multiple segments at the distal end to gradually change the stiffness.

Figure 5. Attain® fixed shape delivery system for CS access. Curve, tip taper, and stiffness profile are designed specifically to aid with cardiac vein sub-selection. Radiopaque tip enhances fluorovisibility.

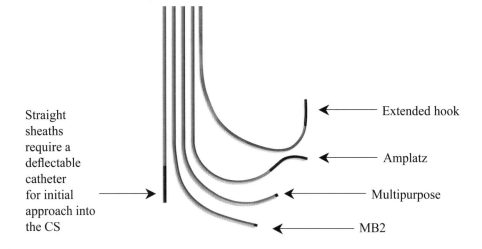

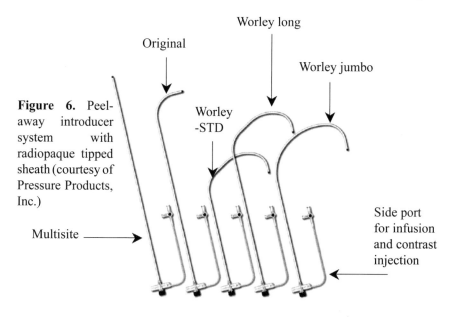

Figure 6. Peel-away introducer system with radiopaque tipped sheath (courtesy of Pressure Products, Inc.)

Figure 7 shows a fluoroscopic image of several catheters (radiopaque tips are more easily viewed).

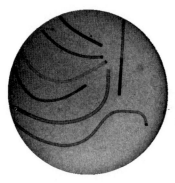

Figure 7. Fluoroscopic view of guiding catheters from different manufacturers.

Other tools are called deflectable catheters. They facilitate CS cannulation in range of cardiac anatomies by allowing the implanting physician to create multiple curve shapes without changing guide catheters (Figure 8).

Figure 8. Deflectable catheter. Rotation of handle offers a variety of curve shapes.

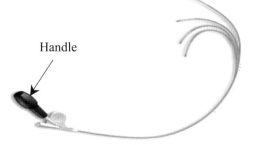

Fixed shapes and deflectable catheters are removed by either pulling apart (peel away or tear away) or cut apart (slittable) along the longitudinal axis of the braided shaft (refer to Figures 9 thru 12 for details).

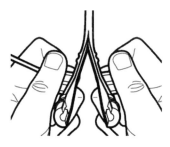

Figure 9. Tear away concept.

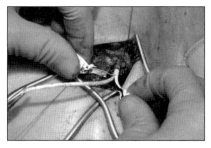

Figure 10. Catheter is gently peeled away while being withdrawn from the vein.

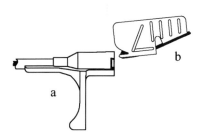

Figure 11. Slittable catheter hub (a) and slitter (b).

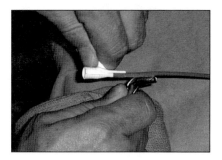

Figure 12. Catheter hub and shaft being cut along longitudinal axis.

There is no mechanism to fix the lead tip into the left heart muscle; instead, most of the LV leads rely on specific distal shapes (angles and curves) to secure their location into a variety of vessels size, tortuosity and angulations. The following figures and sketches illustrate several concepts:

Curves concept (Figures 13 and 14)

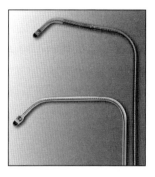 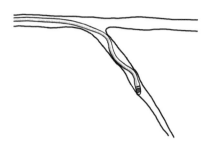

Figure 13. Medtronic Attain™ LV leads.

Figure 14. Attain™ LV lead fixation is achieved by wedging both fixation curves within the cardiac vein.

"S" shaped curve concept (Figure 15)

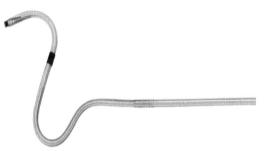

Figure 15. St. Jude Medical Quicksite™ LV lead. The distal preshaped "S" curve presses against the wall of the vein to provide a means of fixation (courtesy of St. Jude Medical).

Straight concept (Figures 16 and 17)

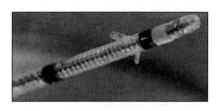 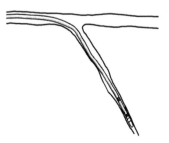

Figure 16. Boston Scientific EASYTRACK® LV lead (courtesy of Boston Scientific).

Figure 17. EASYTRACK® LV lead wedged deep in a vein to find a secure point of fixation (courtesy of Boston Scientific).

"J" shaped curve concept (Figure 18)

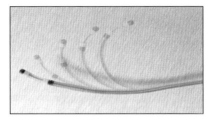

Figure 18. Boston Scientific ACUITY™ LV lead. The J-shaped tip stabilizes the LV lead in the vein (courtesy of Boston Scientific).

Nowadays most of the LV leads are stylet and guidewire (also known as over-the-wire, OTW) compatible. The stylet provides rigidity to facilitate initial venous access. The guidewire helps maneuver into tortuous anatomies and through small and medium-sized cardiac veins. Several lead tip designs have an integrated seal to allow acute guide wire re-insertion and to minimize blood ingress into the inner lumen.

In some cases, the LV lead can be manipulated directly into a suitable venous branch. This method may shorten procedure time and can be tried first if the anatomy seems appropriate based on careful analysis of the CS venogram and morphology of coronary sinus branches. In the case of an acute angled take-off or tortuous venous branch, a 0.014" coronary wire can be advanced into the target vessel and the LV lead is then gently advanced into position (Figures 19 thru 22 illustrate the OTW delivery concept).

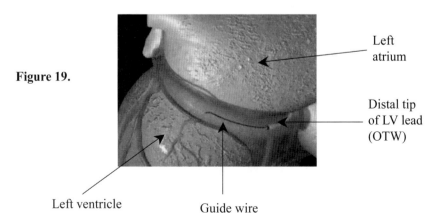

Figure 19.

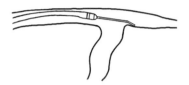 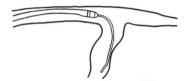

Figure 20. Lead and guide wire advanced near cardiac vein ostium.

Figure 21. Guide wire tip steered deep into the cardiac vein.

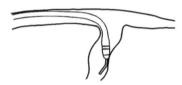

Figure 22. Lead tip is advanced over the wire into the cardiac vein.

Compared with lead implantation for standard pacemakers and implantable cardioverter defibrillators (ICDs), implantation of a specifically designed left ventricular (LV) pacing lead is a relatively demanding procedure. Still, technical advances in delivery systems, availability of multiple LV lead designs, and increased implantation experience of physicians have led to significant decreases in procedural and fluoroscopic times and improvements in overall implantation success rates for CRT systems.

CHAPTER 6

Epimyocardial Lead Terminology and Technology

Epimyocardial pacing is used primarily when transvenous pacing is contraindicated or for patients undergoing concomitant heart surgery. Implant of myocardial/epicardial leads requires an open-chest, tunneling, or minimally invasively subxiphoid approach to attach the lead tip to the outside of the heart (Figure 1).

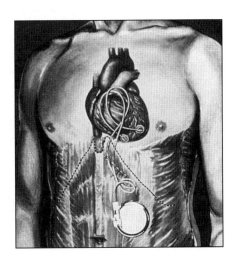

Figure 1. Early pacemaker with myocardial leads.

Construction and components

Stab-in and screw-in leads are considered myocardial leads because they are attached to the outside of the heart and the "hook" electrode and the screw electrode actually pass into the myocardium when fixated. Suture-on leads are considered epicardial leads because the electrode is attached to the outside of the heart and does not penetrate the myocardium (refer to Figures 2 and 3 for definitions and specifics).

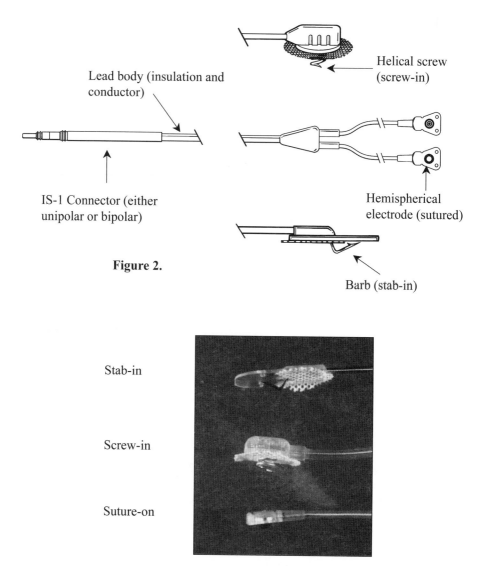

Figure 2.

Figure 3. Examples of epimyocardial lead tip designs.

Components and materials of epimyocardial leads are quite similar to endocardial ones:
- Polarity can either be unipolar or bipolar.
- Silicone and polyurethane are used as prime insulation.
- Conductor mostly made of MP35N.
- Electrodes (with or without steroid) can be used for atrial or ventricular pacing.

Applications

Although the indications for epimyocardial leads are few, they remain an essential mode of pacing therapy for a specific group of patients. They are used in special situations, such as:
- Pediatric applications (the insertion of transvenous pacemaker leads in children is limited by the calibre of the upper chest veins – Figures 4 and 5).
- Congenital malformations.
- When a mechanical heart valve is present.
- Where multiple abandoned endocardial leads are present.
- Concurrent with open-chest surgery.

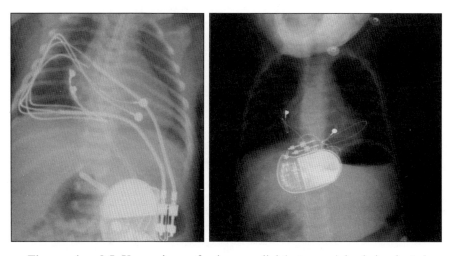

Figures 4 and 5. X-ray views of epimyocardial (suture-on) leads implanted in new-borns.

Special tools required for implant

Implant of a Medtronic screw-in epicardial lead requires the use of a tool to facilitate lead placement (Figure 6). The tool shaft is made up of a malleable material, offering flexibility when placing through endoscope port or rib spreader window (Figures 7 and 8).

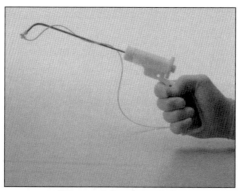

Figure 6. Implant tool.

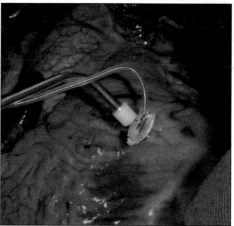

Figure 7. Myocardial screw-in electrode with placement tool.

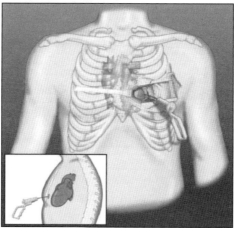

Figure 8. Lateral mini thoracotomy for lead placement.

CHAPTER 7

Temporary Pacing Lead

Temporary pacing leads (also called heart wires) are often attached to the myocardium at the end of the cardiac surgical procedure. Once the leads are placed and connected to an external pacing device, the electrical activity of the heart can be sensed and paced when necessary.

Construction and components

Typical components include a thin curved myocardial needle to minimize trauma during heart wire insertion, one or two electrodes if the construction is either unipolar or bipolar, an insulated conductive wire and a small chest needle (Figures 1 - 4).

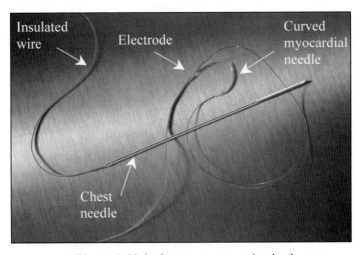

Figure 1. Unipolar temporary pacing lead.

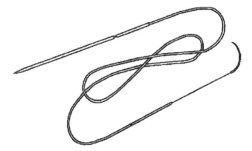

Figure 2. Illustration of a unipolar temporary heart wire.

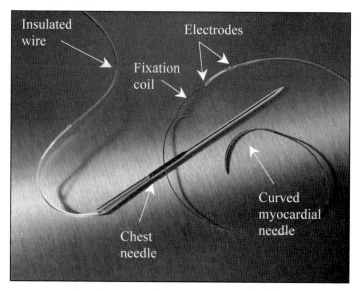

Figure 3. Bipolar temporary pacing lead.

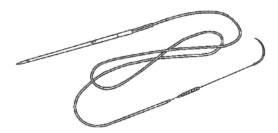

Figure 4. Illustration of a bipolar temporary heart wire.

Chest needles can also be curved. Smaller leads are available and ideal for pediatric patients or small hearts (they include a small fixation coil well suited for thinner pediatric tissue). Several fixation methods are available to anchor the temporary leads in the heart tissue (Figure 5).

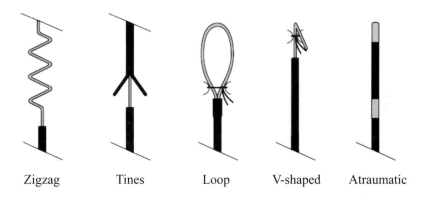

Zigzag　　　Tines　　　Loop　　　V-shaped　　　Atraumatic

Figure 5. Illustration of anchoring methods (courtesy of Osypka).

Applications

Temporary pacing leads are used to support cardiac surgery patients during postoperative recovery, and thus increase the chances of successful surgical outcomes. The leads are placed on the right atrium, right ventricle, or both to restore the conduction system of the ailing heart (Figures 6 and 7). Atrial leads are placed where the muscle is the thickest (the area of the atrium toward the right atrial appendage is thin and may be easily torn by sutures). Ventricular leads are implanted in the surface of the anterior wall of the right ventricle.

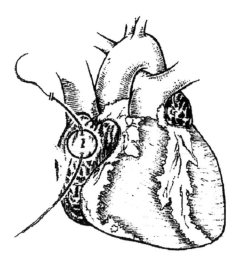

Figure 6. Atrial lead placement.

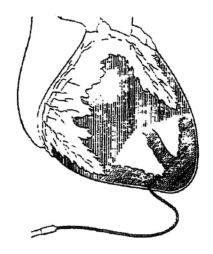

Figure 7. Ventricular lead placement.

Leads are removed 3-7 days post-implant by gently pulling out the wire.

CHAPTER 8

Electrode

The primary purpose of the lead electrode is to act as a long-term interface between the lead and the heart muscle. It is through this interface that the electrical stimulus passes. The other purpose for the electrode is to sense intracardiac signals for the IPG to monitor and to ensure proper pacing when necessary. As such, the electrode must contact the heart in a manner that it is as stable and atraumatic to the tissue as possible and produces minimal inflammatory and fibrotic responses.

Fixation mechanisms

Historically, dislodgment has been one of the most common clinical problems associated with pacing leads. To address this issue, engineers and physicians have responded with a large amount of fixation mechanisms (Figures 1 and 2) to stabilize the electrode, relative to myocardial motion.

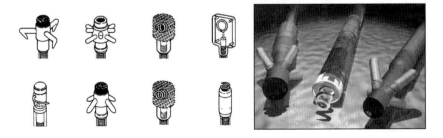

Figures 1-2. Various types of pacing leads with active and passive fixation mechanisms.

Passive anchoring devices, such as flanges or wedge tips and tines were early attempts to solve the dislodgment problems of early pacing leads (Figures 3, 4 and 5).

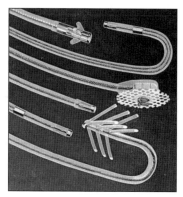

Figure 3.

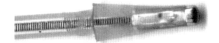

Figure 4.

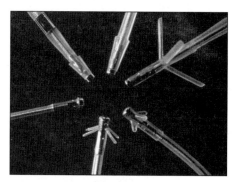

Figure 5.

Passive fixation means that no part of the lead itself is actually embedded in the endocardium; rather, the lead tip is trapped within the trabeculae and/or is held in position by its pre-formed shape (e.g., J-lead in atrium) as illustrated in Figure 6.

Electrode 67

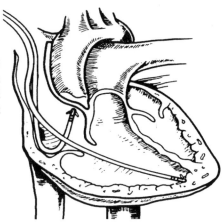

Figure 6. Passive fixation leads with tines. The straight lead is in the right ventricle and the curved lead holds the tip in the right atrium.

Most patients have well-developed trabeculae (Figure 7) in their ventricles and the tines (Figure 8) provide acute and chronic stable electrode anchoring. In the atrium, only the appendage is trabeculated. Therefore, a preformed "J" shaped passive fixation lead is required.

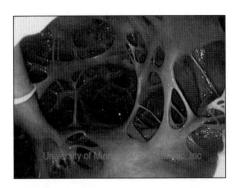

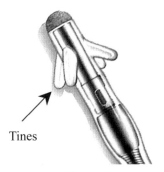

Tines

Figure 7. Trabeculae begin sparsely in the foreground and become much denser within the deep right ventricular apex (courtesy of the University of Minnesota and Medtronic, Inc.)

Figure 8.

Active fixation means that part of the lead actually embeds in the heart tissue for fixation via a screw-in helix electrode. Fixed and extendable/retractable screw-in leads (Figure 9 and 10 respectively) provide excellent stability.

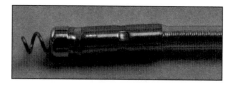

Figure 9.

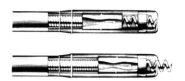

Figure 10. Screw retracted in top view and extended in bottom view. The screw is activated by applying a tool to the connector pin and rotating the inner conductor.

In an extendable/retractable design, the screw is retracted to prevent damage to the veins and cardiac structures during lead advancement and extended for lead fixation. This fixation mechanism is ideal for patients with smooth ventricular walls and for the atrium when the appendage is missing or malformed. These leads are also useful for pacing sites other than the apex of the ventricle or the atrial appendage (e.g. right ventricle outflow tract or septal wall).

Materials and designs

Many electrically conductive materials (such as stainless steel, platinum, platinum-iridium) have been used for the surface material of pacing electrodes. Platinum, platinum-iridium alloy (PtIr 90/10, 80/20 or 75/25 for increased hardness and strength) and activated carbon are used extensively in today's lead electrodes because they exhibit the favorable properties of being corrosion resistant (electrode performance stability is compromised if there is surface corrosion), biocompatible (no toxic or injurious effect).

As illustrated in Figures 11-16, the average geometric surface area of electrodes has decreased significantly thru the last 3-4 decades. Early electrodes had a geometric surface area of over 80 mm^2. Newer electrodes have a geometric surface area of 1.2 to 8 mm^2. This decrease in geometric surface areas has contributed significantly to pacing system efficiency. Ken Stokes (former Medtronic senior research fellow) used the following analogy: "The battery of the pacemaker is like a bucket of water. There is a hole in the bucket, and that represents the current drain through the pacing system electrode. If the hole (electrode) is large, the water (or current) drains out quickly. But if we can make the hole small, then it will drain more slowly."

Similarly, in a pacing lead system, reducing the electrode size increases the pacing impedance (which is the resistance to current flow from the pulse generator to the myocardial tissue) and delivers energy more efficiently (limiting current drain).

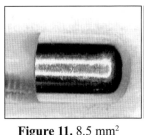

Figure 11. 8.5 mm^2 (1960s)

Figure 12. 8 mm^2 (1970s)

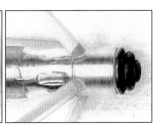

Figure 13. 8.4 mm^2 (1980s)

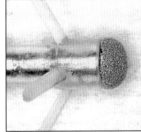

Figure 14. 8 mm^2 (1980s)

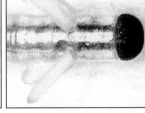

Figure 15. 5.8 mm^2 (late 1980s)

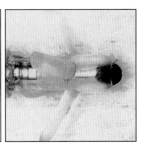

Figure 16. 1.2 mm^2 (mid 1990s)

Unfortunately, simply reducing electrode size is not the final answer; decreased size also increase polarization at the electrode tip due to the smaller surface area (Figure 17).

Figure 17.

Smaller geometric size can increase the impedance but it can also increase the polarization and limit the sensing capability.

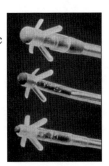

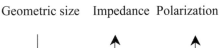

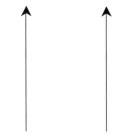

When an electrical current flows, the tip electrode (cathode) attracts positively charged ions. Initially, the movements of these charged ions results in flow of current from the electrode to the myocardium. As the current pulse continues, a charged layer surrounds the tip electrode and produces a capacitive effect. The capacitive effect refers to the build up of a layer of charge on the electrode called polarization (Figure 18).

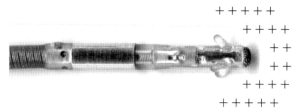

Figure 18. The cathode is negatively charged when the current is flowing, as a result positive ions are attracted at the tip electrode.

When polarization is excessive, a substantial amount of lead current must be used to overcome it and less current is available for simulation of the myocardium. As a consequence, the output voltage must be increased and more lead current is required to maintain an adequate tip electrode voltage and a safety margin.

By altering the surface structure to be more porous, the geometric surface area of the electrode increases and therefore lowers the polarization. Compared to a polished surface, the platinized porous electrodes have a larger functional surface area (Figures 19, 20 and 21 shown at magnification 2,500x).

Figure 19. Polished electrode surface.

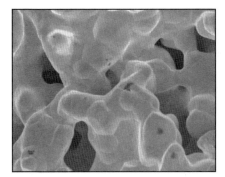

Figure 20. Porous electrode surface.

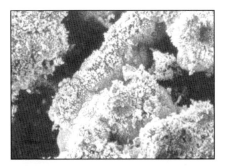

Figure 21. Porous electrode surface.

Surface electrode can also be coated with a thin film of platinum, iridium oxide, titanium nitride or sputtered iridium for even greater surface area as shown in Figures 22 and 23 (magnification 20,000x).

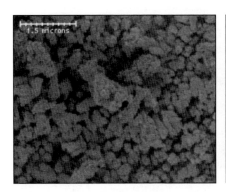 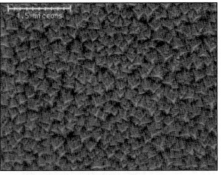

Figure 22. Platinum black.   **Figure 23.** Titanium nitride.

The collective spaces within the electrode pores make up the larger functional surface area, which controls polarization for this geometrically smaller electrode.

In summary, the ideal pacing lead should have an electrode with a small radius (high pacing impedance to increase longevity of IPG) and a large surface area (for good sensing of intrinsic electrical signals from cardiac depolarization and not electrical signals from other sources). The tissue in-growth within the porous structure stabilizes the electrode position (providing a reliable electrode-myocardial contact) which is essential for efficient performance.

From a pacing system efficiency perspective, and as illustrated in Table 1, when the electrode size is reduced, impedance increases leading to lower current drain and improved longevity. Also, when the surface area of the smaller electrode is increased through increased porosity, polarization is reduced, again increasing the longevity of the system.

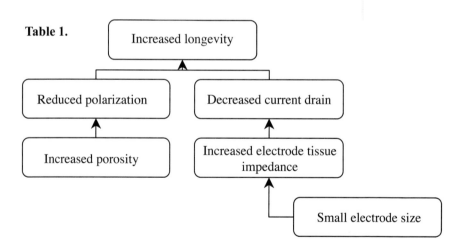

Table 1.

Steroid

A pacing lead is a foreign body that can produce an inflammatory response. Steroid-eluting electrodes provide a continuous elution of dexamethasone (or other corticosteroid) which limits the inflammatory process at the electrode-tissue interface (Figure 24). This benefit can be critically important in children, who typically have a greater inflammatory response to tissue injury and larger threshold rise.

Figure 24. Fewer and less active inflammatory cells congregate at the electrode-tissue site. The illustration compares a steroid eluting lead (top views) to a lead without steroid (bottom views) from the day of implant into the chronic phase. The steroid eluting from the tip of the lead suppresses each stage of the inflammatory process. The result is less inflammation, and a thinner capsule surrounding the lead tip.

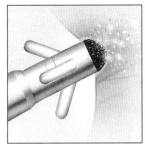
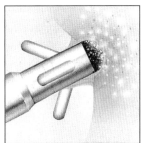
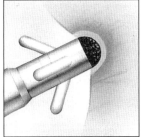
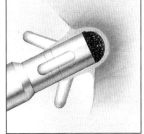

An approach to steroid elution is to coat the electrode (acute benefit) as shown in Figure 25. Another option (chronic elution) is to provide steroid in a reservoir behind the electrode tip (Figure 26) or inside a ring within the distal sleeve (Figure 27). A third approach combines the presence of a reservoir and the coating of the electrode.

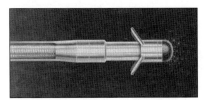

Figure 25. Coated electrode.

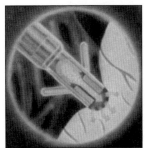

Figure 26. Steroid-eluting reservoir within the electrode.

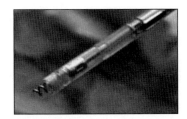

Figure 27. Steroid-eluting ring surrounding the helix electrode.

The steroid is located in the electrode, which is where the lead touches the heart. The very small amount of steroid (less than 1 milligram) is only released into the heart tissue surrounding the electrode. Steroid benefits begin immediately upon implantation. There are published articles from Stokes showing steroid elution over a period of 15 years for tined leads.

Figure 28 illustrates the stimulation thresholds of various type of pacing leads over a 12-week period post-implant. Non-steroid-eluting electrodes exhibit a peaking phase from week 1 to week 5-6, due to the maturation process at the electrode-tissue interface. Steroid-eluting electrodes exhibit virtually no peaking. The chronic phase of stimulation threshold occurs 8-12 weeks post-implant which is characterized by a plateau. This plateau is higher than the acute phase, due to fibrotic encapsulation of the electrode. Steroid-eluting lead chronic thresholds remain close to implant values.

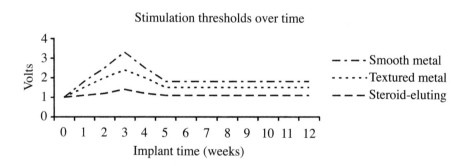

Figure 28.

Stimulation thresholds of steroid-eluting electrodes are kept from peaking in the acute and the chronic periods and therefore extend the pulse generator longevity.

CHAPTER 9

Conductor

The conductor (Figure 1) is a very thin wire that carries electrical impulses from the IPG to the distal tip electrode for pacing or carries intra cardiac signals from the ring electrode to the IPG for sensing.

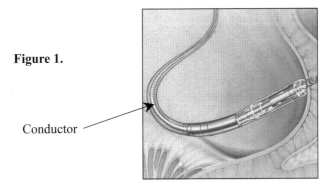

Figure 1.

Conductor

Materials

In 1959, the Swedish electronics firm, Elema-Schönander, and the telecom company, Ericsson, developed a unipolar lead with a conductor that consisted of four thin bands of stainless steel wound around a core of polyester braid (Figure 2). These lead designs were later discontinued because of possible corrosion.

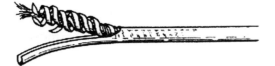

Figure 2. Elema-Schönander unipolar lead with conductor made of stainless steel bands.

Other conductors were made with the drawn brazed strand (DBS) technique (nickel alloy wires drawn together with heated silver – as shown in Figure 3). The polyurethane-insulated leads were found with serious insulation failures caused by internal oxidation from the DBS (corrosion of the DBS) and this type of conductor is no longer used in combination with polyurethane.

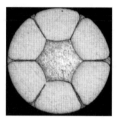

Figure 3. Cross-section of DBS. The silver occupies the central core and the spaces between the nickel alloy wires. Silver also forms a thin coating around the wires.

The tinsel wire (Figure 4) was another early form of electrical conductor. Separated from a central textile core (which provided high tensile strength) the individual strands or ribbons were relatively fragile. The core could also be damaged by high temperature. These two factors made it difficult to terminate the tinsel wire by soldering. Instead, crimped connections were commonly used.

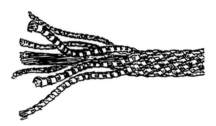

Figure 4. Illustration of platinum/ iridium ribbons intertwined around a polyester yarn.

Today's most commonly used wire is made of MP35N nickel alloy (nominal composition: 35% nickel, 35% cobalt, 20% chromium and 10% molybdenum). It has a low resistance to allow efficient transfer of energy from the pacemaker to the lead tip – thereby helping to minimize energy needed for each impulse from the battery. In addition, it is corrosion-resistant, flexible and durable (Figure 5).

Figure 5. Permanent pacing leads must perform continuously in a very hostile and active environment. The salt content of human blood is similar to sea water (and equally as corrosive). In addition, the lead itself must withstand pressure from bones and ligaments. Plus, at only 70 beats per minute, a lead will flex 100,000 times a day, 37 million times a year, and almost half a billion times in 13 years.

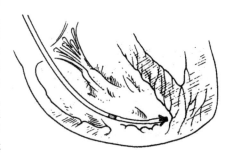

The MP35N silver cored conductor (Figure 6) has the same performance characteristics as the MP35N but offer enhanced conductivity.

Figure 6. Cross-section of silver cored conductor. The inner core can have varying percentages of silver to enhance the conductivity.

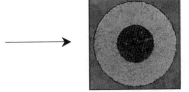

Designs and definitions

A unifilar conductor is a single wire coil that is wound around a central axis in a spiral manner (Figure 7). Coiling the wire helps to facilitate flexibility without breaking.

Figure 7.

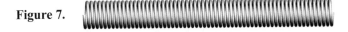

A multifilar conductor consists of two or more wire coils that are wound in parallel together around a central axis in a spiral manner (Figure 8 shows a hexafilar coil construction). This construction helps to reduce impedance in the conductor and builds in redundancy if a filar breaks. Refer to Figure 9 for definitions and characteristics.

Figure 8.

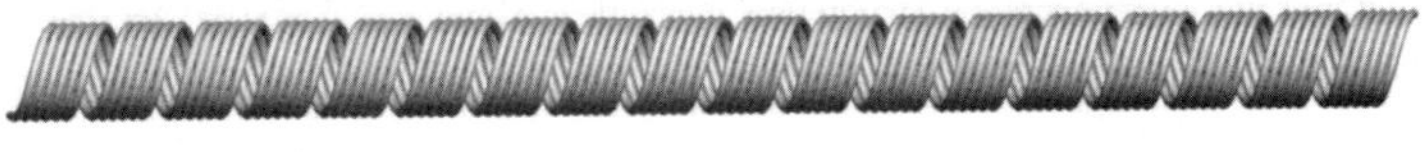

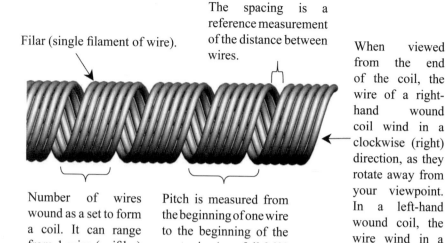

Filar (single filament of wire).

The spacing is a reference measurement of the distance between wires.

When viewed from the end of the coil, the wire of a right-hand wound coil wind in a clockwise (right) direction, as they rotate away from your viewpoint. In a left-hand wound coil, the wire wind in a counterclockwise (left) direction as shown here.

Number of wires wound as a set to form a coil. It can range from 1 wire (unifilar) to 10 (multifilar). Six are shown here.

Pitch is measured from the beginning of one wire to the beginning of the next wire (one full 360° turn). It is calculated by averaging 10 turns of a single wire.

Figure 9.

A cable conductor consists of two or more wires (also called filaments) that are twisted together as a strand and then bundled with other strands around each other like a rope (Figure 10).

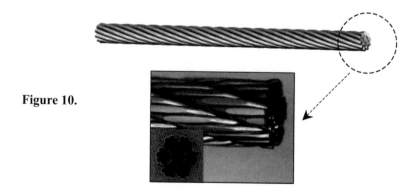

Figure 10.

Coil designs can have good flex fatigue resistance, torsional stiffness, and have a lumen to accommodate a stylet or a guidewire. They have a higher electrical resistance and are more prone to crush failure (first rib-clavicle) compared with cables. Cable designs (many different configurations of filaments and strands are possible) have lower electrical resistance, are less prone to crush and are smaller than coils.

As previously illustrated in this textbook, leads are constructed as unipolar, bipolar or multipolar depending on how many conductors are present to complete the pacing electrical circuit. Today, almost all unipolar leads use multifilar construction with a multifilar coil surrounded by insulation (Figure 11).

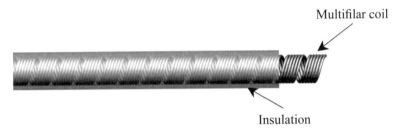

Figure 11.

Nowadays, the most common bipolar lead construction is co-axial where an insulated layer separates two multifilar conductor coils positioned in concentric fashion (Figure 12).

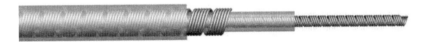

Figure 12.

More complex coaxial lead design can have three conductor coils embedded within concentric layers of insulation as illustrated in Figure 13. This kind of construction was used for tripolar tachy leads.

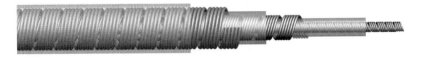

Figure 13.

Other bipolar leads use a coradial construction where two insulated coils are wound next to each other (Figure 14). This design allows the lead body to have a smaller diameter and avoids the complex construction of outer coil and insulation. The engineering challenges are for the coating of the conductors to remain integral along the lead body.

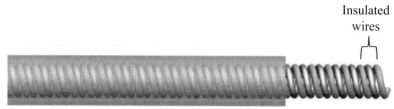

Figure 14.

Some bipolar leads used parallel coil construction as shown in Figure 15.

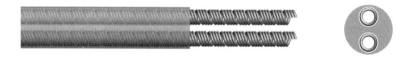

Figure 15.

Modern lead constructions (particularly tachy leads) use a combination of coils and cables (Figure 16). The coil facilitates the passage of a stylet for lead implantation and placement while the cables facilitate a smaller sized lead body.

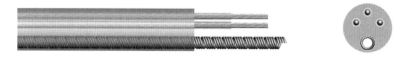

Figure 16.

CHAPTER 10

Insulation

The insulation is a non-conducting material that prevents electrical current from escaping into the tissue surrounding the lead. Insulation also protects the conductor from corrosion due to exposure to body fluids and tissues.

Insulation materials

Silicone and polyurethane are the most commonly used insulation materials in today's pacing leads. Fluoropolymers and copolymers are emerging biomaterials with promising applications in the research and development of future leads.

Silicone

Silicone is a soft and flexible material; it has been introduced since the early days of pacing and continues to be in use today.

<u>Advantages</u>
- Inert (structural composition is chemically inactive).
- Biocompatible (no toxic or injurious effects).
- Biostable (the structure and materials remain relatively unchanged in-vivo).

<u>Disadvantages</u>
- High friction coefficient (the silicone is not inherently slippery and can make difficult venous insertion). Surface processing

techniques can be applied to make the silicone surface more slippery.
- Handling damage (silicone is more prone to damage from abrasion, surface nicks and cuts, attention to handling is imperative - although nicks and cuts can be repaired with medical adhesive).
- Size (some types of silicone leads tend to be larger in diameter than polyurethane leads, because silicone has less tear strength).

Polyurethane

Polyurethane is a firmer, stiffer material than silicone. Compared to a silicone lead, the polyurethane allows for thinner lead body and is also slippery when moist, a helpful attribute when placing two leads in a small vein. Polyurethane (P80A) leads have been implanted in humans since the late 1970s. Because of cases of stress cracking found a few years after, changes in processing were made (elimination of solvents and thermal stress relieving) and subsequent performance has been satisfactory.

Advantages
- Biocompatible (no toxic or injurious effects).
- High tear strength (tougher and resistant to damage by abrasion, surface nicks and cuts).
- Low friction coefficient (they get very slippery in blood by absorbing proteins out of the blood).
- Less fibrotic (the slippery surface reduces platelet adhesion).
- Allows for thinner lead body diameter.

Disadvantages
- Environmental stress cracking (ESC). A crazing or cracking of polyurethane insulation due to the in-vivo environmental exposure in combination with stress. ESC can sometimes result in a complete break or crack through the insulation material. ESC is an oxidative condition that takes place on the surface of polyurethane leads. It initiates on the outside of the lead where

the lead interfaces with the body and propagates inward. It manifests itself by a frosty white surface appearance as shown in Figures 1 and 2.

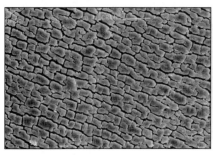

Figure 1. White cracking surface.

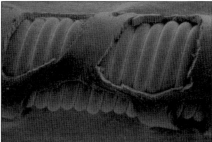

Figure 2. Extreme example of ESC.

- Metal Ion Oxidation (MIO). An oxidative degradation of the polyurethane insulation. Here, the body natural defense against a foreign object produces macrophage cells that produce peroxides. The peroxides migrate through the polyurethane and the oxygen molecules from the peroxides mix with the metal ions from the conductor. This mixture works to oxidize the polyurethane as shown in Figures 3 and 4.

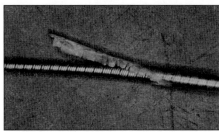

Figure 3. Insulation has completely oxidized and broken away from the left side of this lead.

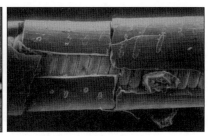

Figure 4. MIO of inner insulation.

A stiffer polyurethane (known as 55D) is used more commonly today than P80A because it is much less susceptible to ESC.

Fluoropolymers

Fluoropolymers (PTFE – polytetrafluoroethylene, and ETFE – ethylenetetrafluoroethylene) are utilized primarily as a coating to protect conductor wires from corrosion and can serve as redundant insulation.

Advantages
- Inert (structural composition is chemically inactive).
- Biocompatible (no toxic or injurious effects).
- High tensile strength (strong, firm material allowing small sizes).

Disadvantages
- Stiff. Most silicone and polyurethane insulations average between 0.007" and 0.010" in thickness. At this same thickness PTFE and ETFE are too rigid and are much thinner for lead applications.
- Fluoropolymers are prone to developing pinholes (which make the lead susceptible to MIO) during the manufacturing process.
- Susceptible to creep (they flow under stress).

Copolymers

Silicones are known to be biostable and biocompatible in most implants, they have the low hardness and low modulus useful for many device applications. Conventional silicone elastomers can have very high ultimate elongations, but only low to moderate tensile strengths. In contrast, conventional polyurethane elastomers have excellent physical properties. They combine high elongation and high tensile strength. The prospect of combining the biocompatibility and biostability of the silicone elastomers with the processability and toughness of polyurethane is an attractive approach to what appears to be a nearly ideal biomaterial.

Optim™ lead insulation is a copolymer used on St. Jude Medical cardiac leads. It is a material that blends the biostability and flexibility of silicone and the durability and abrasion-resistance of polyurethane. As indicated by St. Jude Medical, Inc. (which has an exclusive license for use of the material), the copolymer has the following characteristics:

- Improved lubricity (in bench testing, SPC showed less frictional value than silicone or polyurethane).
- Improved flexibility (in bench testing, lead tip stiffness was considerably less stiff than 55D polyurethane and similar to silicone rubber).
- Increased abrasion-resistance (in normalized bench test data, the lead insulation was more resistant to abrasion in 'lead-on-lead' contact testing than silicone rubber).
- Stability (after two years of implantation, the material has shown biostability at least as good as 55D polyurethane).

Note: Elast-Eon® and SPC indicate early development names for Optim™ insulation. Elast-Eon® was designed at the Commonwealth Scientific and Industrial Research Organization (CSIRO) in Melbourne, Australia, as a biostable material for use in life-critical medical devices. Elast-Eon is a trademark of Aortech.

PurSil™, manufactured by the Polymer Technology Group (PTG), is another thermoplastic polyurethane-silicone copolymer material. In addition to possessing silicone in the polymer backbone, the PurSil™ material contains polymer chains that are also terminated with silicone Surface-Modifying End Groups™ (SME).

The PurSil™ 35 copolymer contains approximately 35% silicone (by weight). It has been suggested that the covalently bonded silicone protects the polyether soft segment from oxidative degradation in vivo. This biomaterial may combine the biocompatibility and biostability of silicone with the processability and tensile strength of polyetherurethane.

Properties of insulation materials

Implanted transvenous leads are subjected to a variety of loading forces which may lead to insulation damage. Insulation material should be flexible, durable, and have low friction.

In the device pocket, the insulation may be exposed to compressive forces at sites where the lead contacts itself, another lead body, or the IPG. Compression set and abrasion can occur in this region.

- Compression set is the permanent deformation of a material after being subjected to compressive forces over time. Compression set is usually manifested by localized areas of thinning in the lead insulation (Figure 5). In a pacing lead, this can occur where the lead is wrapped against itself under the IPG or between the first rib and clavicle.

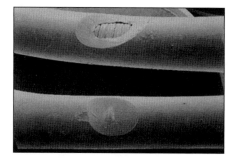

Figure 5.

- Abrasion is the rubbing off or wearing away of material caused by frictional forces of one body sliding over another (Figure 6). This can happen when two leads rub against one another or when bone or ligaments are in a position to constantly rub against a lead.

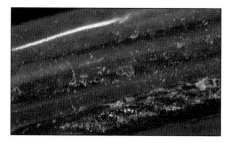

Figure 6.

In the region of the first rib and clavicle (Figure 7), cyclic compression (crush) may result in disruption of the insulation (Figure 8).
- Crush is resistance to rupture as a material is compressed between two objects.

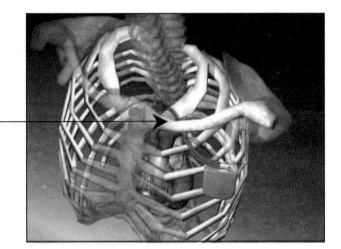

Figure 7. First rib and clavicle region.

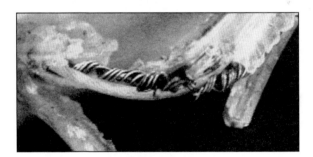

Figure 8.

In the area where the lead passes into the heart from the superior vena cava the lead is subject to elongation and creep as it responds to the beating heart.
- Cold flow is a time-dependent dimensional change (usually thinning as shown in Figures 9 and 10) due to movement or flow of a polymer under load.

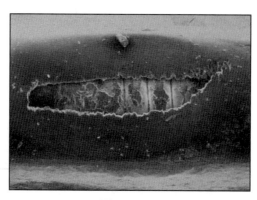

Figure 9.

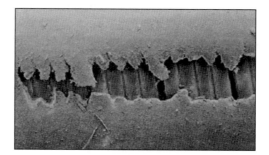

Figure 10.

- Elongation is the amount of stretch that occurs before a material breaks.

CHAPTER 11

Connector

The connector forms a junction between the pacing lead and the IPG (Figure 1). An accurate mechanical fit between the connector and the cavity of the pulse generator is crucial for the safe transmission of current from the pulse generator without current leakage.

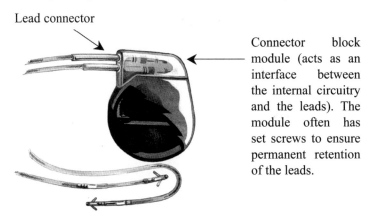

Lead connector

Connector block module (acts as an interface between the internal circuitry and the leads). The module often has set screws to ensure permanent retention of the leads.

Figure 1. Illustration of the connection between the proximal end of the pacing lead to the connector block of the pacemaker. A tight fit seals out body fluids and completes the conduction pathway.

Designs and definitions

Pacing leads connectors have significantly changed over the last decades (Table 1). Early designs (5/6 mm unipolar, as shown in Figure 2, and bifurcated bipolar connectors) evolved into in-line 3.2 mm connectors (also known as low profile). In-line designs brought a lot of confusion and problems for the implanting physicians since some manufacturers placed the sealing rings on the connector while others had them placed inside the connector block of the IPG.

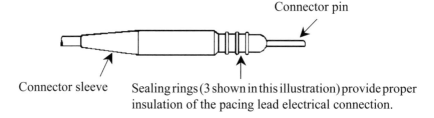

Figure 2. Illustration of a 5/6 mm unipolar connector.

Because of this lack of standardization and incompatibility between system components, manufacturers agreed on a VS-1 and IS-1 configurations which include sealing rings on the proximal portion of the lead. VS-1 is a Voluntary Standard while IS-1 is a formal International Connector Standard (ISO 5841-3) developed jointly by the International Organization for Standardization and the International Electrotechnical Commission in 1992, whereby pulse generators and leads so designated are assured of a basic mechanical fit.

Table 1.

Connector description	Illustration of design
Bifurcated bipolar 5/6 mm	
Unipolar 5/6 mm	
Low profile 3.2 mm – no sealing rings	
Low profile 3.2 mm with sealing rings	
IS-1 and VS-1	

Current unipolar and bipolar IS-1 lead connectors are 3.2 mm in diameter, have sealing rings, a short connector pin and offer a great uniformity. Unipolar connectors have a blue connector ring as a visual indication that the lead is unipolar. The leads are labeled IS-1 UNI (Figure 3) or IS-1 BI.

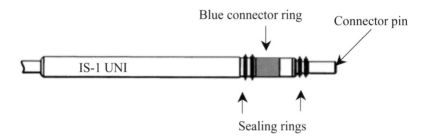

Figure 3. IS-1 unipolar connector.

Adaptors

A major challenge for manufacturers of leads and pacemakers has been the compatibility between lead connectors and connector block modules. It is a significant concern when approaching a patient for a pulse generator replacement.

The compatibility can be achieved by using a lead connector that matches the configuration of the IPG connector block. Another option is to use an adaptor to upsize or downsize the lead connector and the sealing mechanism to fit the connector block. Figures 4, 5 and 6 show various examples of adaptors and their applications.

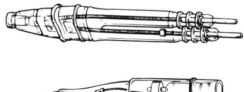

Figure 4. Adaptor to connect a 3.2 mm bipolar lead to a bifurcated bipolar IPG connector block.

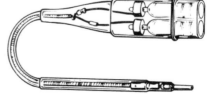

Figure 5. Adaptor to connect a 5 mm bifurcated bipolar lead to a 3.2 mm bipolar IPG connector block.

Figure 6. Adaptor to connect a 3.2 mm low profile bipolar lead to an IS-1 bipolar IPG connector block.

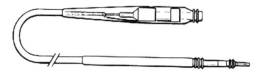

Adaptor kits may also include medical adhesive (silicone) and wrenches as shown in Figure 7.

Figure 7. Adaptor with wrenches.

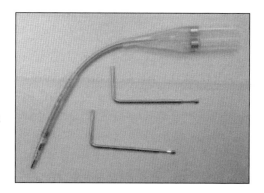

CHAPTER 12

Stylet and Guide Wire

Stylet

Stylets provide additional stiffness and controlled flexibility for maneuvering the lead into position. They vary in length (although matching the lead measurement), stiffness and shape to accommodate the physician's preference for lead and stylet flexibility (Figures 1 and 2 and Table 1). Stylet diameter is in the typical range of 0.014" to 0.016".

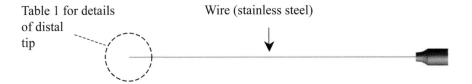

Figure 1. Straight stylet.

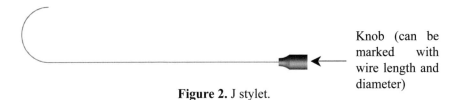

Figure 2. J stylet.

Table 1.

Distal end	Illustration of distal shape
Blunt	
Ball-tipped	
Extended taper, ball-tipped	

When it comes to implanting an atrial J-lead (preformed J-shape), a straight stylet will ease the initial insertion and movement thru the veins. Once in the right atrium, the stylet is pulled out and the lead resumes its J-shape for positioning in the atrium.

Stylets can also be bent (specific curves and planes) to position a straight active fixation leads into selective sites (i.e. right ventricular outflow tract as illustrated in Figure 3).

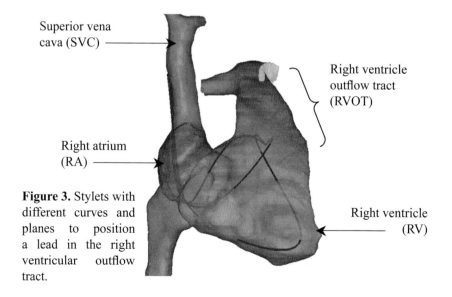

Figure 3. Stylets with different curves and planes to position a lead in the right ventricular outflow tract.

Stylet guide

A stylet guide is intended to ease the insertion of a stylet into the connector pin of the lead (Figure 4).

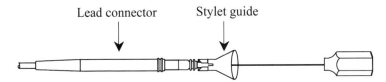

Figure 4. Use of a stylet guide to facilitate stylet insertion.

Locking stylet

Extraction of chronically implanted leads is facilitated by using specialized locking stylets. To avoid breakdown of the lead during traction, a locking stylet (Figure 5) is introduced into the central lumen. It consists of a straight wire with a locking mechanism that can be secured within the inner coil close to the distal end of the lead. The tensional force exerted via the locking stylet is almost directly delivered to the tip, limiting unwanted stretching of the lead body while establishing a firm rail over which extraction sheaths can be maneuvered. Locking mechanisms differ between manufacturers and recently introduced devices can be unlocked and repositioned if necessary.

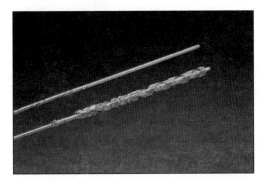

Figure 5. LIBERATOR® locking stylet (courtesy of Cook Medical, Inc. / Cook Vascular, Inc.)

Guide wire

0.035" J-tipped guide wires are part of the accessories used in support of initial venous access during a lead implantation. The soft "J" configuration facilitates advancement through tortuous venous systems while minimizing inadvertent trauma to the structures. Commonly made of stainless steel, they can be treated with a hydrophilic coating, they vary in length (45 to 180 cm) and offer various tip curve radius (Figure 6).

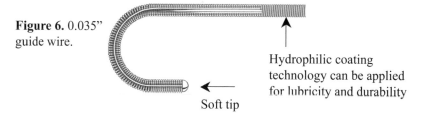

Figure 6. 0.035" guide wire.

Hydrophilic coating technology can be applied for lubricity and durability

Soft tip

Soft 0.035" guide wires can be used with guiding catheters to cannulate the coronary sinus (CS) ostium (during left ventricular lead implantation). Figure 7 illustrates a 0.035" guide wire ahead of a delivery catheter before further advancing the catheter into the CS.

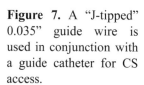

Figure 7. A "J-tipped" 0.035" guide wire is used in conjunction with a guide catheter for CS access.

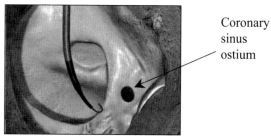

Coronary sinus ostium

Guide wires (generally 0.014" diameter) can also provide support and trackability for placement of the over-the-wire (OTW) left ventricular leads (Figure 8). The most distal zone is sufficiently floppy to prevent trauma to the vessel walls through which the guide wire and lead are inserted (Figure 9). An intermediate zone is generally stiffer and the third zone is stiffer yet. Lubricious coatings are also provided to reduce friction between the lead and guide wire.

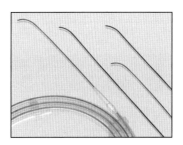

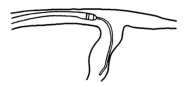

Figure 8. Soft 0.014" guide wires.

Figure 9. Illustration of a guide wire tip steered deep into a cardiac vein.

CHAPTER 13

Suture Sleeve

The suture sleeve (also known as anchoring sleeve) is a small grooved tube-like component that fits around the body of a lead to secure the lead in place (Figure 1). Sleeves are made of silicone rubber which can also be mixed with barium sulfate (radio-contrast agent for X-ray imaging).

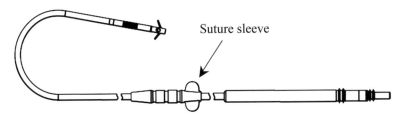

Figure 1. Suture sleeve located at the connector end of the lead.

Some suture sleeves include a single groove (Figures 2 and 3), multiple grooves (to give implanting physicians more choices when anchoring the lead) and tabs (Figures 4 and 5). They are used to secure the lead from moving and to protect the lead insulation and conductor coil from damage caused by tight ligatures.

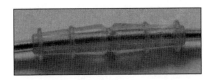

Figure 2.

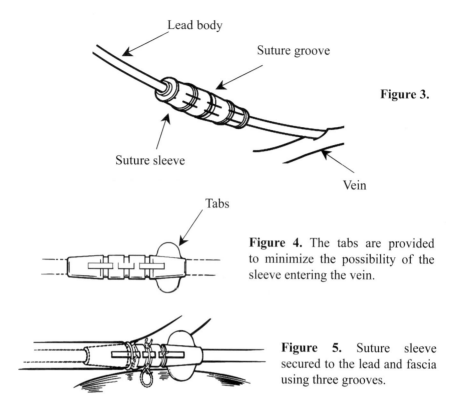

Figure 3.

Figure 4. The tabs are provided to minimize the possibility of the sleeve entering the vein.

Figure 5. Suture sleeve secured to the lead and fascia using three grooves.

Coil fracture and/or insulation failure at or around the site of introduction into a vein accounts for a significant number of lead failures. The suture should be tied to prevent the lead from moving within the sleeve, but not too tight that it might deform the lead conductor coil (Figure 6). Suture cannot be tied directly to the lead body.

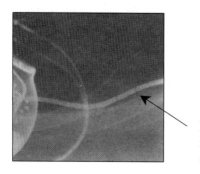

Figure 6. Visible distortion indicating excessive tightening around the suture sleeve.

CHAPTER 14

Fluorovisibility

Equipment

The imaging system is an important prerequisite for implantation and verification of lead positioning. The equipment can be portable (Figure 1) or fixed but must be able to provide antero-posterior (AP – as shown in illustration below) and oblique views to confirm specific target implant sites.

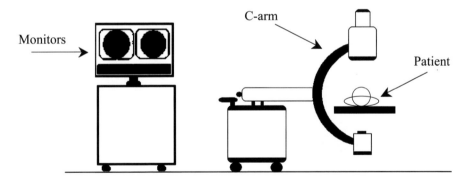

Figure 1. Fluoroscopic imaging system.

Views and interpretations

In an AP view the fluoroscopic imaging system is positioned directly above the patient, the sternum and the spine are in line (Figure 2).

Spine

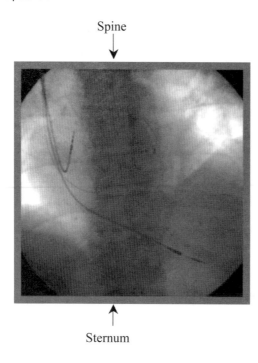

Figure 2. Anteroposterior view. Spine and sternum are in line. Ribs curve away from the spine with the same angulation on both sides.

Sternum

In a right anterior oblique (RAO) view, the equipment has been moved to the right of the patient and the sternum is to the right of the spine (Figure 3).

Spine

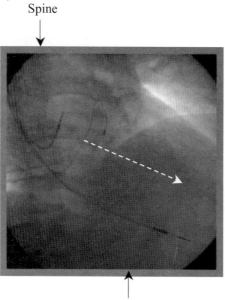

Figure 3. Right anterior oblique. The sternum is to the right of the spine. The ribs can be seen sloping downward as shown by the arrow (negative slope).

Sternum

In a left anterior oblique (LAO) view, the system is on the left of the patient and the sternum is to the left of the spine (Figure 4).

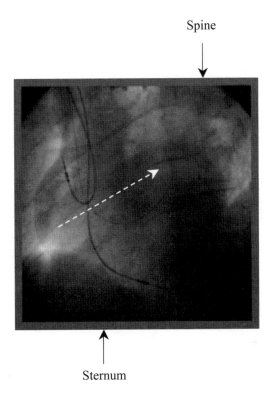

Figure 4. Left anterior oblique. The sternum is to the left of the spine. The ribs can be seen sloping upward as shown by the arrow (positive slope).

Visual quality can vary widely among different fluoroscopy units and techniques. Plastics and less dense materials are not visible in fluoroscopy. Denser metals, such as platinum, are more easily viewed.

Distal portion of leads are shown under normal fluoroscopic conditions in Figures 5, 6 and 7.

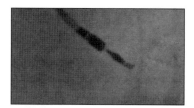

Figure 5. Bipolar active fixation.

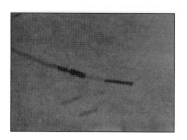

Figure 6. Bipolar passive fixation.

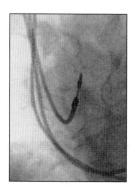

Figure 7. Bipolar J active fixation.

When active fixation leads are implanted, fluoroscopy is used to verify helix electrode extension and/or retraction. Figures 8 and 9 illustrate possible views and interpretations (which vary among manufacturers). Image magnifier will be helpful to visualize the details.

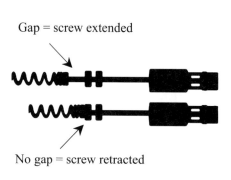

Figure 8.

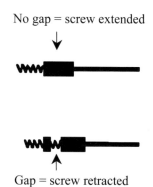

Figure 9.

Glossary

Active fixation lead A pacemaker or defibrillator lead with a screw-like mechanism at the tip that attaches to the inner surface of the heart.

Acute threshold The threshold measured at time of initial implantation.

Adams-Stokes syndrome A condition characterized by sudden transient attacks of lightheadedness or unconsciousness, with or without convulsions, due to a temporary cessation of blood supply to the brain. It is named after two Irish physicians, Robert Adams (1791-1875) and William Stokes (1804–1877).

Adaptor A special connector used between an otherwise incompatible implantable pulse generator and a lead.

Alternate site pacing Cardiac pacing at a site of the heart other than the conventional pacing sites (ventricular apex or atrial appendage).

Ampere (A) The unit of electric current (current is abbreviated i or I).

Anchoring sleeve A small grooved tube-like component that fits around the body of a lead to secure the lead in place (also called suture sleeve).

Anode In a bipolar lead it is the proximal band (also called ring electrode or band electrode).

Antitachycardia pacing (ATP) A therapy for treating ventricular tachycardia that consists of the rapid delivery of sequences of pacing pulses to terminate the arrhythmia.

Apex The blunt extremity of the heart formed by the left ventricle.

Appendage A structure arising from the surface or extending beyond the tip of another structure.

Arrhythmia Any variation from the normal rhythm of the heartbeat.

Atrial appendage A small muscular pouch attached to each atrium of the heart.

Atrium One of the two upper chambers of the heart (plural: atria).

Beats per minute (BPM) The unit of measurement of heart rate.

Biocompatibility The quality of not having toxic or injurious effects on biological systems.

Biostability The ability of a material to maintain its physical and chemical integrity after implantation in living tissue.

Bipolar lead A lead that has a conductor leading to the tip electrode (cathode) and a second conductor leading to the ring electrode (anode).

Biventricular pacing A system designed to restore contraction synchronization of the left and right ventricles (also called cardiac resynchronization therapy).

Bradycardia A cardiac arrhythmia which refers to a slow beating of the heart (under 60 beats per minute).

Brady lead A lead through which an IPG delivers impulses (also called low-voltage lead or bradycardia lead).

Can The metal shell of an implantable device (IPG or ICD).

Capacitor Electronic component within an ICD which stores an electrical charge.

Capture The ability of an electrical discharge to cause stimulation of the myocardium.

Cardiac cycle A complete cardiac movement, or heart beat, including systole, diastole, and intervening pause.

Cardiac output The volume of blood pumped by the heart per minute.

Cardiac resynchronization therapy (CRT) Any therapy delivered by a class of devices that is designed to assist the mechanical function of the failing heart, by stimulating a more coordinated biventricular contraction.

Cardiomyopathy A disease of the heart muscle that causes it to become enlarged and lose strength to pump blood.

Cardioversion therapy A high voltage therapy (synchronized to a ventricular sensed event) for termination of a tachycardia.

Catheter A tubular, flexible, surgical instrument that is inserted into a cavity of the body to withdraw or introduce fluid, or to introduce a flexible device.

Cathode The distal electrode in both a bipolar and a unipolar lead.

Chronic threshold The threshold of a pacing system that has been implanted for some time.

Coaxial lead design A lead that has a conductor in the center, a circumferential outer conductor, and an insulating medium separating these two conductors. The outer conductor is also insulated.

Coil electrode A flexible electrode at the distal end of a tachy lead used to deliver high voltage shocks (coil electrode can either be located in the superior vena cava and/or in the right ventricle).

Coradial lead design A lead in which the conductor is made of individual wires separately insulated and then wound together in parallel into a single coil. This construction allows for a thinner lead body.

Conductor A thin wire that transmits electrical impulses from the pacemaker to the electrodes.

Connector The portion of a pacing lead that is connected to the pacemaker.

Connector block module The part of an implantable pulse generator into which the leads are plugged (also called header).

Connector pin A hardware feature designed to allow electrical flow from a lead or wire to a device.

Connector sleeve A small grooved tube-like component that fits around the body of a lead to enable mechanical and electrical connection.

Coronary sinus A collection of veins joined together to form a large vessel that collects blood from the myocardium of the heart.

Crimp sleeve A small metal cylinder used to join components by mechanical compression.

CRT-D An ICD enabled with Cardiac Resynchronization Therapy (CRT).

CRT-P An IPG enabled with Cardiac Resynchronization Therapy (CRT).

Defibrillation lead A cardiac lead, either transvenous or patch, which acts as part of the electrical system in conjunction with other leads or the can electrode to provide defibrillation therapy.

Defibrillation therapy A therapy consisting of an electrical shock to terminate a ventricular fibrillation. The ICD attempts to synchronize the shock to a ventricular depolarization, and if unsuccessful, delivers the shock asynchronously.

Defibrillation threshold (DFT) The minimum amount of energy required to defibrillate the heart.

Dexamethasone A steroid used to reduce acute cellular trauma.

DF-1 The international standard for a unipolar connector between an implantable defibrillator lead and an implantable cardioverter defibrillator.

Diastole The time period when the heart is in a state of relaxation and dilatation (expansion).

Drawn brazed strand (DBS) Alloy wires stranded around a core wire of a softer, highly conductive material such as silver.

Ejection fraction (EF) A measure of how well the heart pumps blood.

Electrocardiogram (ECG or EKG) A graphic representation of the electrical activity of the heart, as recorded by surface electrodes.

Electrode The portion of a pacing lead that acts as a long-term interface between the lead and the heart tissue.

Electrode-tissue interface The area of complex interaction between the pacing lead active electrode and the heart tissue.

Endocardium The innermost layer of tissue that lines the chambers of the heart.

Environmental stress cracking (ESC) A crazing or cracking of polyurethane insulation due to the in-vivo environmental exposure and internal stress.

Epicardium The outer layer of heart muscle.

Epimyocardial lead A type of pacing lead designed to be attached to the outside of the heart. Helical and barb designs make contact with the epicardium but pass into the myocardium when fixed, hemispherical electrode designs make contact with the epicardium but do not penetrate the myocardium.

ETFE Ethylenetetrafluoroethylene.

Fibrillation Quivering or spontaneous contraction of individual muscle fibers.

Fluoroscope A device used to project a radiographic (X-ray) image on a fluorescent screen for visual examination.

French A unit of measure of diameter.

Guidewire A wire or spring used as a guide for placing a larger device.

Heart block A condition in which impulses are not conducted in the normal fashion from the atria to the ventricles.

Heart failure (HF) A condition that is characterized by the buildup of fluid in the lungs or in other parts of the body.

Helix electrode A spiral-shaped structure at the most distal end of a lead used for lead fixation.

High impedance lead A pacing lead with a reduced electrode size which increases the pacing impedance value, thereby reducing current drain.

Impedance The total opposition to current flow in a pacing system (the term resistance applies only to idealized circuits with constant voltage and current and no capacitors). Expressed in Ohms (Ω).

Implantable cardioverter defibrillator (ICD) An implantable device that detects and treats tachyarrhythmias, providing antitachycardia pacing, bradycardia pacing, cardioversion, and defibrillation therapies. The device is sometimes called automated implantable cardioverter defibrillator (AICD)

Implantable device A manufactured product that is inserted into the human body and is expected to stay there for 30 days or more.

Implantable pulse generator (IPG) The portion of a pacing system that produces electrical impulses. It contains the power supply (battery) and the electronic circuitry (also called pacemaker).

In vivo Refers to experimentation done in or on a living tissue.

Indifferent electrode An electrode dispersing electrical stimulation over a large area.

Integrated bipolar An ICD lead with an anode integrated into the right ventricle coil electrode.

Insulation A non-conducting material that prevents electrical current from escaping into the tissue surrounding the lead.

Introducer sheath A tubular, flexible instrument that is used to introduce another flexible device, such as a cardiac lead or a balloon catheter, into the body through blood vessels.

IS-1 The international standard for a bipolar or unipolar connector.

IS-4 The international standard for a quadripolar connector.

Isodiametric Having the same diameter in all directions.

Lead The portion of a pacing system that contains conductor, insulation, electrode and connector to connect to the pacemaker.

Lead body The insulated main or central part of a lead.

Lead maturation process A period beginning at lead implantation during which myocardial stimulation thresholds begin at low voltages, rise, and decline to a plateau.

Lead pin cap An accessory used to seal the end of a pacing lead which is no longer in use.

Left-heart lead A lead that is specifically designed to pace the left ventricle. It is placed through the coronary sinus and then into the branch cardiac veins.

Metal induced oxidation (MIO) An oxidative degradation of the polyurethane insulation.

MP35N A nonmagnetic, nickel-cobalt-chromium-molybdenum alloy possessing a unique combination of ultrahigh tensile strength, good ductility and toughness, and excellent corrosion resistance.

Myocardium The muscular tissue (middle and thickest layer) of the heart.

New York Class Association (NYHA) Classification A system of classifying heart failure patients into one of four categories (class I, II, III or IV) depending on their symptoms and functional capacity.

Ohm (Ω) The unit of electric resistance (abbreviated R).

Pacemaker cardioverter defibrillator (PCD) A name given to the first implantable cardioverter defibrillator.

Pacing threshold The minimum amount of energy (or battery power) needed to make the heart beat consistently.

Passive-fixation lead A pacemaker or defibrillator lead that uses appendages of insulation material, such as tines, at the tip.

Patch lead A type of cardiac electrical lead that is attached to an ICD on one end and to the heart's surface on the other.

Polarization The build up of opposing electric charges on the surface of an electrode.

Polarization resistance The resistance to flow of electrical current by polarization of positive ions moving toward the negative electrode and negative ions moving toward the positive electrode. It is time-related and the resistance increases as more ions migrate.

Polymer A substance containing a large number of structural units joined by the same type of linkage.

Polyurethane A polymer consisting of a chain of organic units joined by urethane links. Polyurethane is used as an insulating material on a lead.

PTFE Polytetrafluoroethylene.

Residual torque A twisting force on the inner conductor of an active fixation lead that remains after the helix is extended.

Ring electrode An electrode that surrounds the lead body near the distal tip.

Screw-in lead A lead with a helical tip that is attached to a tissue using a clockwise motion.

Selective site pacing Cardiac pacing at any specific, unconventional site of the heart such as the atrial septum, ventricular septum, right ventricular outflow tract, or bundle of His.

Silicone A polymer that has a "backbone" of silicon-oxygen linkages. Silicone is used as an insulating material on a lead.

Steroid A drug that reduces inflammatory response (especially useful at the electrode-tissue interface).

Stylet A thin, shapable wire that runs through a lead to stiffen its body during implantation.

Subclavian crush Damage to a pacing lead caused by compression of the lead between the rib and the clavicle (also known as clavicle/first rib entrapment).

Systole The time period when the heart is contracting (specifically during which the left ventricle of the heart contracts).

Tachy lead A lead through which an ICD delivers shocks (also called high-voltage lead or tachycardia lead or defibrillation lead).

Tachycardia A cardiac arrhythmia which refers to a rapid beating of the heart (greater than 100 beats per minute).

Telemetry A technology that allows the remote measurement and reporting of information.

Temporary lead A lead intended for short term use which is placed either epicardially after open heart procedures or transvenously, and is usually connected to an external pacemaker.

Tensile strength The force required to pull a material to the point where it breaks.

Thoracotomy An incision into the chest to gain access to the thoracic organs, most commonly the heart, the lungs, the esophagus or thoracic aorta.

Threshold The minimum stimulus required to cause excitation of the myocardium.

Titanium nitride (TiN) A compound of titanium and nitrogen that adds surface to an electrode.

Transvenous Through a vein or through the venous system, as in the passage of a device or catheter through a vein for diagnostic or therapeutic purposes.

Unipolar lead A transvenous unipolar lead has a conductor leading to the tip electrode (cathode).

Venogram A method of visualizing blood vessels by injecting a contrast medium into a vein prior to performing an X-ray.

Ventricle One of the two lower chambers of the heart.

Volt (V) The unit of electrical potential (abbreviated V).

X-ray Penetrating radiation similar to light, but having much shorter wavelengths. They are usually generated by bombarding a metal target with a stream of high-speed electrons.

Xiphoid process A small fragment of cartilage located at the lower end of the sternum (also called xiphisternum).

Suggested Readings

- Bakken E. *One Man's Full Life.* Medtronic (1999).
- Barold S, Mugica J. *The Fifth Decade of Cardiac Pacing.* Blackwell Publishing (2004).
- Barold S. Stroobandt R, Sinnaeve A. *Cardiac Pacemakers Step by Step.* Blackwell Publishing (2004).
- Ellenbogen K, Kay N, Wilkoff B. *Device Therapy for Congestive Heart Failure.* Saunders (2004).
- Ellenbogen K, Wood M. *Cardiac Pacing and ICD's.* Blackwell Publishing (2005).
- Gras D, León A, Fisher W. *The Road to Successful CRT Implantation. A Step-by-Step Approach.* Blackwell Futura (2004).
- Hayes D, Lloyd M, Friedman P. *Cardiac Pacing and Defibrillation: A Clinical Approach.* Blackwell Publishing (2000).
- Hayes D, Wang P, Sackner-Bernstein J, Asirvatham S. *Resynchronization and Defibrillation for Heart Failure. A Practical Approach.* Blackwell Futura (2004).
- Iaizzo, P. *Handbook of Cardiac Anatomy, Physiology, and Devices.* Humana Press (2005).
- Kenny T. *The Nuts and Bolts of Cardiac Pacing.* Blackwell Futura (2005).

Suggested Readings

- Kenny T. *The Nuts and Bolts of ICD Therapy.* Blackwell Futura (2006).
- Kenny T. *The Nuts and Bolts of Cardiac Resynchronization Therapy.* Blackwell Futura (2007).
- Lüderitz B. *History of the Disorders of Cardiac Rhythm.* Futura (2002).
- Mond H., Karpawich P. *Pacing Options in the Adult Patient with Congenital Heart Disease.* Blackwell Futura (2007).
- Moses W, Miller B, Moulton K, Schneider J. *A Practical Guide to Cardiac Pacing.* Lippincott Williams & Wilkins (2000).